1

Time Bomb

A Survivor's Story of Recovery from Multiple DVTs
and an Underlying Aortic Aneurysm

Kim McDonell

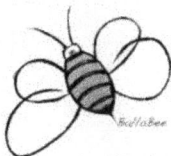

Don't wait for the boom, learn the signs with *Time Bomb* and save a life.

Disclaimer

I am not a doctor, or a medical professional of any kind.

This book details my personal experience of the origins, symptoms, diagnosis, surgery and recovery from an aneurysm on my ascending aorta. Nothing contained herein is medical advice, or may be construed as a substitute for medical advice.

If you have concerns about your health, you MUST consult a qualified medical doctor.

Aneurysm

An aneurysm is a bulge in the wall of a weakened blood vessel.

An aneurysm can occur anywhere in the body.

Rupture can be fatal.

Contents

Chapter 1

Background

It was a calm and sunny day when I decided to take my darling two-year-old son Jason, to his first toddlers' morning at Tubrid Church. Excitement filled the air as we arrived at the church, looking forward to meeting new mums and toddlers for some fun.

The morning turned out to be everything we expected and more. Jason was giggling and playing, making new friends, and experiencing the joy that only toddlers can bring. As the event concluded, we said goodbye to our newfound friends, ready to head back home and continue our day.

Little did I know that a life-changing event was just around the corner. As we journeyed home in my trusty Toyota Celica, a car carrying newlyweds rushing to catch their honeymoon flight, skidded towards us. Hidden by a hedge and a turn in the road, their approach was unseen until the moment of impact.

In that split second, as chaos unfolded around me, something within urged me to bring my car to a stop. Instinctively, I reacted by shifting my gears to neutral, a decision that would prove to be crucial and taking my foot off the brakes. It's difficult to explain the source of that inner voice, but I listened intently as it guided my actions. I let go of the wheel and lunged across to protect my infant son.

The forceful collision sent my car spiralling into a surreal state of slow motion. The steering wheel bore the brunt of my chest impact, and everything seemed to move in a blur. My thoughts raced as I tried to comprehend what had just happened, struggling to process the shock and fear coursing through my body.

Soon after, the authorities arrived at the scene, lending their assistance and expertise. However, the swelling in my voice box prevented me from communicating effectively. All I could do was remain calm, relying on their guidance and support to navigate the aftermath of the crash. On the small narrow road we had been travelling on, another car approached and the driver corroborated my limited account of events.

As the police commenced their investigation, it became evident to them that the fault lay mainly with the speeding honeymooners, not me. From the length of the skid, their excessive speed was calculated to be a dangerous 70 miles per hour. The evidence spoke for itself, validating that it was indeed the other driver's recklessness that had led to this disastrous collision.

In that harrowing moment, it felt as though the world had come to a standstill. The incident had shaken me to my core and left me grappling with emotions and unanswered questions. But as I reflect on that fateful day, I can't help but feel an overwhelming sense of gratitude for the unseen force that urged me to take evasive action and prevent a potentially catastrophic outcome. I take it as a testament to the importance of listening to one's instincts.

While the crash left its mark physically and emotionally, I am eternally grateful that my son, Jason, was safely secured in his car seat, facing the rear of the car. This precaution undoubtedly played a vital role in protecting him from harm. It is a reminder of the unpredictability of life and the fragility of our existence.

I will always be grateful for the professionalism and efficiency of the Police, who, when I couldn't speak for myself, were able to read the evidence for the truth. Justice prevailed, ensuring that our lives could move forward with a newfound appreciation for each precious moment we share.

With three broken ribs and a swollen voice box, I embarked on a 16-year journey in search of the pain over my heart that never seemed to go away after this unforgettable day in the year 2000. I was 30 years old and this event would become a turning point in my life, reminding me to cherish every breath, every precious second, and hold my loved ones just a little tighter.

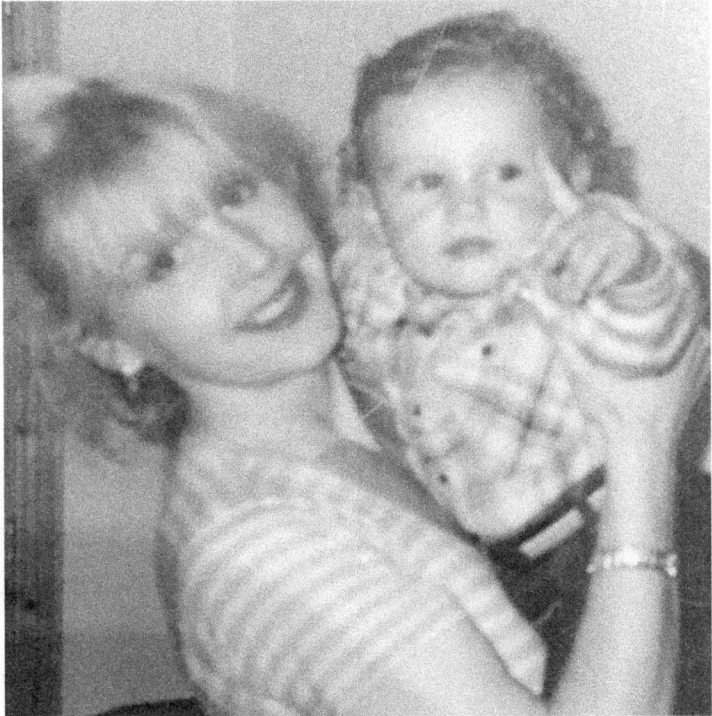

Jason and I around the time of the accident

Chapter 2
Mexico 2002

On a beautiful Christmas Day in 2002, I had the once-in-a-lifetime opportunity to swim with dolphins in Mexico. The setting was idyllic, with crystal-clear turquoise waters and a vibrant sun shining above. Excitedly, I waded into the water, thrilled at the prospect of interacting with these magnificent creatures.

As soon as I entered the water, one dolphin in particular, called Hermes (I remember as it's also the name of a designer brand) seemed unusually attentive to me, swimming around and occasionally nudging me towards the edge of the enclosure. At first, I thought it was just playing, enjoying the interaction. However, the instructor, well-versed in dolphin behaviour, approached and informed me of a remarkable possibility.

He explained that dolphins have an exceptional ability to sense things beyond human perception. This particular dolphin, by repeatedly pushing me towards the edge, was attempting to communicate something quite extraordinary. The instructor believed that the dolphin somehow sensed an underlying illness, even though I was completely unaware of it myself.

Little did I know, a potentially life-threatening blood clot was forming in my leg at that very moment. Remarkably, this perceptive creature picked up on the presence of a hidden danger. Dolphins, known for their intelligence and intuition, can detect changes in energy and subtle cues. This extraordinary ability, combined with their affinity for humans, allows them to form remarkable connections with people, transcending language barriers.

Although I couldn't understand the dolphin's warning signals at the time, looking back, it fills me with awe and gratitude. It serves as a powerful reminder of the profound connection we can share with these incredible creatures.

Swimming with dolphins that day turned out to be an enlightening and almost otherworldly experience. Not only did I witness their playful nature and grace, but I also became profoundly aware of the keen instinctive capabilities they possess. It is a day forever etched in my memory as an insight into the fascinating allure of dolphins and their extraordinary connection with humankind.

Returning home to Belfast after the unforgettable experience of swimming with dolphins in Mexico, I was plagued with excruciating pain in my leg. I entered the Royal Victoria Hospital with deep concern and uncertainty as my left leg was swollen, throbbing and burning. The smell of antiseptic greeted me, reminding me of the seriousness of the medical environment. After checking in and patiently waiting, my name was called, and I was led to a cramped yet efficient examination room.

The doctor explained the importance of conducting a Doppler imaging scan, a non-invasive diagnostic procedure that uses sound waves to see the blood flow in my leg. Concerned and curious, I agreed to undergo the scan, hoping that it would shed some light on what was causing the pain and discomfort. Lying on a narrow table, I watched as the technician gracefully manoeuvered the ultrasound device across my leg. The room was dimly lit, calming nervousness as a sense of anticipation filled every corner. With each swish of the ultrasound probe and each cross-section of my leg appearing on the monitor, a subtle tension built within me. As the scan progressed, the images on the screen revealed the truth that had remained hidden within my body. The doctor's face turned serious, hinting at the severity of the discovered clot in my left leg. The imaging clearly showed the obstruction in a deep vein, disrupting the normal blood flow.

It was then, in that medical room, that I learned for the first time about the presence of a blood clot that posed a grave risk to my health. The diagnosis brought a mix of emotions - relief for discovering the cause of my discomfort, fear for the potential implications, and gratitude for the timely intervention.

The medical team swiftly began arranging a treatment plan of Warfarin therapy that kept my blood thin. They explained the importance of immediate action to prevent further complications. The gravity of the situation sank in as I understood the impact this blood clot could have had if left undetected. The urgency of the medical attention was clear and underlined the importance of listening to our bodies and the subtle warnings they often send.

Leaving the Royal Victoria Hospital a week later, a newfound awareness occupied my thoughts. The remarkable incident in Mexico, where the perceptive dolphin had repeatedly nudged me towards the edge of the enclosure, now held an even deeper significance. This unexpected encounter with the dolphin had unknowingly acted as a curious precursor to my rendezvous with the medical world, ultimately leading to early detection and timely treatment.

The experience at the Royal Victoria Hospital marked the beginning of a journey towards recovery. It would be the same place that I would return to 14 years later with the root cause of my clots.

Chapter 3

Summers on the Farm with Auntie Moira

As the summer holidays approached, anticipation and excitement welled up within me. For as long as I can remember, these precious weeks were filled with joy, adventure, and unforgettable experiences on Auntie Moira and Uncle Barry's lively farm. From the ages of 6 to 13, I found myself eagerly returning each year, delighting in the wonders of farm life.

Upon my arrival, the farm buzzed with activity and welcomed me with open arms. Turkeys and Ducks waddled by quacking away to one another, as chickens pecked at the ground, cooing with contentment. Pigs, with their endearing snouts and curly tails, became instant favourites, captivating me in the most enchanting way. I found sheer delight in watching the sows nurturing their litters of piglets and witnessing the tender moments shared between mother and child.

Among the lively menagerie, two characters stood out from the rest - lovable goats named Dolly and Daisy. Their mischievous spirits and playful antics brought moments of pure entertainment and laughter. Dolly had a peculiar fondness for clothes, particularly when they were hung on the washing line. Many times, I caught her nibbling on the colourful garments that swayed in the gentle breeze. My aunt, always resourceful, would salvage the bits of fabric Dolly managed to devour for her patchwork quilts, incorporating these unexpected contributions into vibrant masterpieces. Spending time with Dolly became a cherished part of my farm experience. We would embark on adventures exploring the vast expanse of meadows and woodlands. Dolly's dainty hooves danced across the uneven paths, as I followed closely behind, the patchwork quilt of memories growing with each step.

But the farm was more than just a place of bustling activities and wonderful animals. It served as a sanctuary, a haven where love and family flourished. The bonds formed with Auntie Moira and Uncle Barry grew stronger with each summer visit. Their patience, guidance, and support taught me invaluable life lessons, shaping my character and nurturing my soul.

As I reflect on those cherished summers spent on the farm with Auntie Moira, I am reminded of the abundance of love and joy that weaved its way through every moment. The timeless memories created, the friendships forged, and the connection to nature and animals that grew within me - all of these continue to be a heartfelt reminder of the simple, wholesome pleasures that we too often overlook in the humdrum of everyday life.

Ah, the vivid memory of the day Auntie Moira entrusted the farm to my care still brings a mix of amusement and embarrassment. It was a gloomy day, with raindrops gently tapping against the farmhouse windows. Auntie Moira and Uncle Barry had left to attend a neighbour's funeral, about a mile away, leaving me responsible for my younger cousins William and Elizabeth.

Thinking I could handle the responsibility, I decided it would be a great idea to take our two mischievous goats, Daisy and Dolly, for a walk on dog leads. Now, in hindsight, that may have been the start of my downfall. With William and Elizabeth eagerly joining me, we set off for what I thought would be a leisurely stroll around the farm.

Little did I realise, as we strolled down the lane that met the road, that the funeral procession was passing by at that very moment. The sight of our two goats ambling alongside us, their leads held securely in our hands, caused quite a commotion among the mourners. To my horror, I found myself nearly smack in the middle of the solemn event, oblivious to the grief-stricken faces directed at our peculiar parade.

Thankfully, the goats sensed my panic (I think!) and decided it was the perfect time for some antics of their own. With a sudden burst of energy, they tugged at their leads, leading us on an impromptu sprint up a nearby hill, away from the funeral and the indignant whispers that followed in our wake.

When Auntie Moira and Uncle Barry returned, I knew instantly that I was in for a scolding. Auntie Moira's face was a mix of fury and worry as she learned of our escapade. She exclaimed words I won't repeat here, but they were fuelled by the love and genuine concern she had for us.

Looking back now, it's clear how reckless and foolish my decision was. Auntie Moira's anger was justified, as she trusted me with the safety of William and Elizabeth. It was a valuable lesson; it taught me to think before acting, and to never underestimate the unpredictable nature of goats on dog leads! That day remains a memorable reminder of the reckless innocence of childhood, alongside the guidance and patience of Auntie Moira. Though she may have scolded me then, her love for me remained, just as her farm where cherished memories, both mischievous and tender, will forever remain in my heart.

Over the years, my Mother, a nurse, has wondered aloud where my talent for sewing, creating beautiful furniture, and love of animals came from. As I reflect on my past, I can attribute a significant portion of these passions to Auntie Moira, my Mum's sister. She played a vital role in inspiring my creativity and ultimately led me to start my own successful interior design business. She possessed a unique talent for sewing, designing intricate patchwork patterns and creating templates out of cornflake boxes to create perfect diamonds, squares and circles for her fabric to mould into amazing patchwork quilts. Her inventive spirit pushed the boundaries of what was considered conventional, and she continually sought new ways to express herself through her creations.

Being in Auntie Moira's presence was an immersive experience. She taught me the joy of using my hands to transform simple materials into extraordinary works of art. With patient guidance and encouragement, she cultivated my skills and nurtured my creative instincts. Although Auntie Moira's time with us was limited, the impact she had on my life endures.

One of the most valuable lessons that Auntie Moira imparted was the importance of thinking 'outside the box'. She believed that the solutions to life's challenges often lay beyond the obvious. She encouraged me to explore alternative paths and embrace the unexpected in my search for answers. Auntie Moira's influence kindled a fire within me, igniting a desire to constantly push boundaries and pursue my passions with tenacity and an open mind.

Spending summer holidays alongside my cousin Elizabeth, it was evident that we possessed different inclinations. While Auntie Moira's daughter devoured books with an insatiable thirst for knowledge, my interests leaned more toward the lively world of farm animals. Though we were kin, it seemed that Elizabeth and I were forged from different particles of the universe.

As children, we would often spend time together at Auntie Moira's house. Elizabeth, never parting with a book, would curl up in a cosy corner, her nose buried in pages filled with fantastical adventures. I, on the other hand, would wander outside to explore the farm and discover the joys of tending to animals.

As I navigated life's twists and turns, I found solace in Auntie Moira's teachings. Her belief in the power of creativity and her ability to find beauty in the mundane inspired me during difficult times. Whether I faced personal dilemmas or encountered obstacles in my professional pursuits, I would draw from the well of Auntie Moira's wisdom, striving to adapt and find innovative ways to overcome challenges. Looking back, it's clear that Auntie Moira's spirit lives on within me. Her legacy is not only reflected in my artistic endeavours but also in the compassion and love I hold for animals. Auntie Moira had a deep connection with nature and instilled in me the importance of caring for and understanding the creatures that share our world.

Elizabeth's love for reading was infectious. She would regale me with tales of daring heroes, magical creatures, and far-off lands, painting vivid pictures within my imagination. Though I had a fondness for farm animals, her passion was undeniable, and I found myself drawn to her enthusiasm.

One sunny afternoon, as we sat beneath the shade of a sprawling oak tree, Elizabeth handed me a book. It was a tale of animals on a farm, a gentle bridge connecting our different worlds. I delved into the story, and with every turn of the page, I discovered the fascinating lives of the animals that I so fondly cared for. As the farm animals took on personalities, engaging in their adventures within the pages before me, I developed a newfound appreciation for Elizabeth's love of reading. Through her eyes, I began to understand the magic that lay within books – the power to transport us into new realms, pique our curiosity, and broaden our understanding of the world. Elizabeth and I often found ourselves merging our interests, creating imaginative tales where farm animals embarked on grand quests, using their unique talents to overcome obstacles. In these shared narratives, our worlds intertwined, forming a beautiful blend of literature and nature.

And so, as Elizabeth and I journeyed through life, our paths may have diverged, but the memories and lessons we shared would forever remind us of the intertwined bond we forged. We remained bookworm and lover of farm animals - different but bound together by the resounding echoes of Auntie Moira's presence and the love of storytelling that brought us closer, chapter by chapter. It was within the pages of countless books that I found revelation and understanding, as I navigated the quest to find the root cause of my heart pain. The wisdom and insights gleaned from literature became my guide, unravelling the layers of my pain and leading me towards healing. In this way, my passion for reading, ignited by Elizabeth and her love for books, became instrumental in my search for answers and brought me closer to understanding the complexities of my own heart.

In our fast-paced and ever-changing society, Auntie Moira's lessons of thinking outside the box remain as relevant as ever. Her memory serves as a constant reminder to approach life's hurdles with creativity and a willingness to explore uncharted territories of possibility.

My sense of identity is growing stronger as I type. I realise that I am not just an individual wandering through life; I am part of a lineage bound by talents and dreams. The talents of Auntie Moira, and perhaps other ancestors, have taken root within me, guiding my creative endeavours and shaping the contours of my soul.

Amidst the beauty of Auntie Moira and Uncle Barry's farm, there existed an unexpected connection to the exhilarating world of motorcycle racing. In a small cottage nestled just up the road, Joey Dunlop - the legendary TT racer - resided with his wife and children. Joey, being a second cousin to Uncle Barry, brought an air of excitement and thrill to the ordinary countryside. Where tractors and machinery melded with the idyllic landscape, Joey's cottage served as a beacon of adventure. It was surrounded by an aura of speed, risk, and the unmistakable aroma of motor oil. In those humble surroundings, the legendary racer witnessed his family grow, with his baby son Gary, still a toddler, adding a sense of innocence to the otherwise adrenaline-charged atmosphere.

My fascination with Joey's daredevilry began to bloom from a young age, and as I grew older, I became more determined to experience the thrill of riding on his powerful motorcycle. Each summer break, I'd muster all the courage within me and pester Joey relentlessly, pleading for that one ride that would fulfil my dreams. Finally, he gave in and took me for a ride that I would never forget.

We embarked on our journey, zipping through idyllic country roads, the wind whipping through my hair and a triumphant grin stretching across my face. With each bend we took, the world became a blur of vibrant colours and fleeting landscapes. The speed at which Joey piloted the bike was nothing short of breathtaking, leaving me with a mix of awe and exhilaration.

As we approached a particularly sharp turn on Burnquarter Lane, the bike leaned heavily, testing the limits of physics and my courage in equal measure. I clung to Joey, trusting in his skill and experience as the lean angle grew more extreme. Suddenly, my knee grazed the road and my dungarees tore open as a trophy of the adventure in progress. After that wild ride on the back of Joey's bike, I made a firm decision never to ask him for another spin. The experience had pushed me well beyond my comfort zone, and the fear it instilled in me overshadowed any sense of excitement or adventure.

Surviving the ride felt like a blessing, and it made me realise that this kind of exhilaration was simply too far outside of my boundaries. The lack of control during the journey was a stark reminder of the risks involved. I couldn't help but be grateful to be back on solid ground and in one piece. From then on, I chose to prioritise my safety and well-being over the lure of thrills and new experiences. While the ride had certainly been fun, I couldn't disregard the valuable lesson it taught me about knowing and respecting my limits. Thank you to Joey the TT Legend.

Dolly, the mischief-maker, had an insatiable appetite for Uncle Barry's striped shirts. It was an unfortunate snack choice, but in the world of quirky coincidences, it led to a welcome turn of events for my beloved dungarees. Little did I know that this choice would weave a thread of connection to Auntie Moira's magical talents. Oh, Auntie Moira, the queen of transforming misfortunes into beautiful patches, had a knack for creating art out of unexpected odds and ends. Her patchwork masterpieces were truly one-of-a-kind, filled with stories and memories that would forever make me smile at my dungarees.

In that moment, as I chose to fashion my dungaree patch from Uncle Barry's striped shirt, I couldn't help but feel a wave of Auntie Moira's creativity wash over me. It was as if she whispered in my ear, encouraging me to think laterally and take the path less travelled.

Dolly's snack-induced mishap symbolises for me the beauty of the unique and the serendipity of the unexpected; a reminder to choose options that defy conventional norms, to embrace the endless possibilities that lie behind door number three or four, or any other unexplored path.

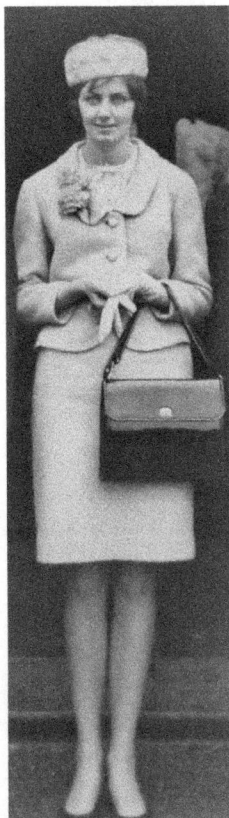

Oh, how time flies and life can take unexpected turns. In the year 2000, Auntie Moira delivered devastating news - she was diagnosed with cancer. It was a heartbreaking blow to our family, and sadly, she passed away in 2002. Her absence left a void within us all, but her memory remains etched in our hearts.

Driven by a deep desire to honour Auntie Moira's artistic legacy, I embarked on a journey to China in 2004, searching for a factory that could replicate her beautiful patchwork designs. Auntie Moira's patchworks were true works of art, painstakingly crafted over months and enriched with her passion and creativity. However, in China, there were factories capable of producing them at a faster pace, without compromising on quality. It was a bittersweet realisation, knowing that Auntie Moira's intricate labour could be replicated in a shorter time frame.

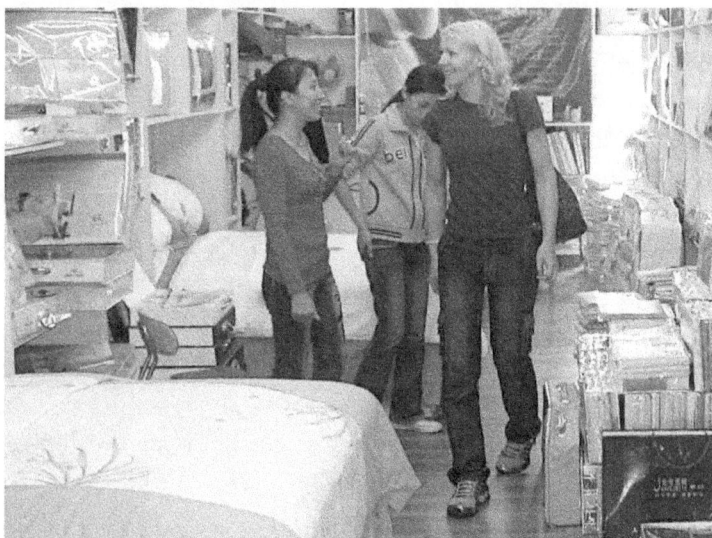
Visiting a Commodity Market in China

Arriving at Beijing Airport, on the way to the baggage reclaim I came across a Chinese foot and body masseuse catering to weary arrivals - something of a novelty to Western travellers but taken very seriously by the Chinese. By applying pressure to different parts of the feet, a skilled massage therapist can identify pressure points and use foot reflexology techniques to alleviate tension throughout the body.

Thrilled by the prospect of experiencing a wonderful massage on my sore legs after a long flight, I settled into one of the plush leather chairs and prepared to relax. My anticipation was short-lived, however, as the Chinese lady providing the massage abruptly halted her actions when she reached a certain point on my left leg. At the time, I assumed she simply did not wish to focus on massaging my legs. It was only later, upon my return to Ireland, that I discovered she had detected a deep vein thrombosis (DVT). Thankfully, my treatment only entailed a six-month course of Warfarin.

Despite this revelation, I remained perplexed as to the cause of the recurring pain over my heart area every time I undertook a long-haul flight.

Oh, the discomfort and pain that accompanied me on those journeys! I knew then there was more wrong inside me than doctors could explain. But with each setback and hardship, I found strength in preserving Auntie Moira's legacy and bringing her artistic creations to life. While China provided an opportunity to continue her patchwork traditions, it was also a journey mired in poignant memories and personal struggles. It is times like these that remind me of the transient nature of life and the importance of cherishing those we hold dear. Auntie Moira's talent, her patchwork masterpieces, and the memories we shared remain with me as reminders of her creative spirit and the beauty she brought into my life.

Chapter 4
USA, 2009

In 2009, I went on an exciting trip to the United States with Ewan and Jason. The adventure began when we flew from Belfast to Newark, New Jersey. With my past experiences in the back of my mind, I wore compression socks during the long flight to America. At that time, I still knew nothing about the underlying condition that may have made the use of compression socks ineffective.

The trip included many thrilling experiences. One memory that stands out is the time we decided to go to Carowinds amusement park, near Charlotte. As we slid down the log flume, I felt my heart racing, almost bursting with pain. Fortunately, Jason didn't want to go on any of the rollercoasters at the park, bringing an early end to the day's adventures that could have turned into tragic consequences for me.

Another memorable experience during my USA trip was jet skiing on Lake Norman. It was exhilarating, but I didn't know at the time that this fun-filled memory would be tinged with pain later on. If I had been aware of my aneurysm, I would have chosen to avoid engaging in activities that could potentially put me at risk. Unfortunately, wearing compression socks on the flight over would not have been enough to mitigate the risks associated with an aneurysm.

Despite these incidents, I continued to make the most of my time in the United States, exploring various destinations and creating lasting memories. However, as the trip progressed, I began to experience persistent pain and discomfort in my leg.

After returning to Ireland, I sought medical attention at the Erne Hospital in Enniskillen. It was during a Doppler ultrasound scan that the presence of another blood clot was discovered. I was prescribed Warfarin again, along with an anticoagulant medication to prevent clot formation and further health complications. Adhering to the treatment plan and continuing regular medical checks became crucial in managing my condition effectively.

Looking back, my trip to the USA in 2009 brought both joy and unexpected health challenges. It reinforced the significance of listening to my body and recognising potential risks associated with certain activities. The subsequent medical care and treatment I received played a vital role in addressing the blood clot and reducing the risk of future complications.

What I know now: an aneurysm on the ascending aorta refers to a weakened or bulging section on the large blood vessel that carries oxygenated blood from the heart to the rest of the body. In my case, blood was pooling or stagnating within this bulging section, which increased my risk of clot formation.

During long-haul flights, individuals with an aortic aneurysm may be at an increased risk of developing clots due to several factors: Firstly, long periods of immobility, such as sitting in cramped aeroplane seats, can lead to slowed blood flow and pooling of blood in the lower extremities. This stagnant blood creates an environment more prone to clot development.

Secondly, the reduced cabin pressure and lower oxygen levels in an aeroplane's cabin can contribute to the formation of clots. These conditions may lead to a heightened state of hypercoagulability (thicker blood) and increased platelet aggregation (clumping together) in some individuals.

Thirdly, the combination of immobility and dehydration during long flights may further increase the risk of clot development. Reduced movement can hinder blood from flowing freely, while dehydration can cause blood to become more concentrated, increasing its likelihood to coagulate and form clots.

If a clot forms within the aneurysm during a long flight, the consequences can be serious. The clot can obstruct or partially block blood flow, potentially leading to further complications such as aneurysm rupture, organ damage, or even stroke if the clot breaks off and travels to other parts of the body.

To minimise the risk of clot formation during long-haul flights, individuals with aortic aneurysms should consider taking preventative measures. This may include staying well-hydrated, frequently moving and stretching within the confines of the aeroplane, wearing compression stockings to aid blood circulation, and consulting with a medical professional for personalised advice, including any necessary blood-thinning medication.

Individuals with an an aortic aneurysm must be aware of their condition and the associated risks, and take necessary precautions, particularly during activities such as long flights that can potentially impact their health. It's always best to consult with a healthcare professional who can provide specific guidance based on individual circumstances.

Moving forward, it is essential for me to continue monitoring my health closely, following medical advice, and making necessary lifestyle adjustments to maximise my well-being and minimise the chances of future complications.

Chapter 5
France 2015

In the beautiful summer of July 2015, Ewan and I embarked on a memorable trip to France, accompanied by our son Jason and his girlfriend Rachel. Excitement filled the air as we set off on an adventure to immerse ourselves in the rich culture and breathtaking landscapes of this captivating country.

As the plane glided through the clouds, an excruciating pain intensified within my chest, causing an overwhelming sense of panic. Each breath became a challenge, and thoughts of mortality clouded my mind. Fearful and uneasy, all I wanted to do was lie down in the aisle to get away from the torment.

Upon landing in France, a sense of urgency pushed me to seek help immediately. Determined to find relief, I hastened to a nearby local chemist. Thankfully, luck was on my side as the French chemist I encountered spoke English fluently, alleviating the language barrier that existed due to my limited French proficiency. I can sing Frère Jacques, but that's about it!

Anxiously explaining my condition to the chemist, I conveyed the immense pain I had experienced during the flight, describing it as originating from over my heart. Displaying concern and professionalism, the chemist evaluated my symptoms and began considering potential solutions.

After some thought, the chemist suggested a magnesium taurate supplement, highlighting its various potential uses, including those associated with heart-related conditions. Expounding on the possible benefits, I learned that magnesium taurate is a form of magnesium, an essential mineral known for its role in various bodily functions, especially within the cardiovascular system.

The chemist explained that magnesium taurate might help regulate heart rhythms, support optimal heart muscle function, and reduce the risk of certain cardiovascular ailments. It is commonly thought beneficial for individuals experiencing heart-related irregularities or discomfort, potentially providing the relief I had so fervently sought.

Intrigued by this potential solution, I eagerly took the suggested magnesium taurate supplements. As I did, a flicker of hope kindled within me, accompanied by gratitude for the knowledge and expertise of the French chemist.

Throughout the remainder of our trip, the magnesium taurate supplements became a staple in my daily routine. Their effects gradually unfolded, and with each passing day, the pain that had plagued me during the flight started to fade. The gentle alleviation of discomfort coupled with the astounding beauty of France allowed me to fully appreciate the wonder and joy of exploring this captivating country.

While we were there, a scorching heat wave swept across the country, leaving us sweltering and eager for the cool of the shade. At the time, we didn't know it was unusual – it was the height of summer, and we thought that it was normal for that time of year. Delighted and intrigued by the beauty around us, we found sanctuary in the exotic garden of our stunning rented villa in Seillans. With its sprawling pool and inviting outdoor kitchen equipped with a barbecue area, the villa seemed like a paradise, providing both relaxation and distraction from the pain of the Time Bomb I was to discover in months to come.

As the sun beat down relentlessly, our days were filled with a delightful mix of rest and exploration. We revelled in the refreshing waters of the pool, seeking respite from the sweltering heat. Laughter and joy permeated the air as we soaked up the sun's rays, cherishing every precious moment spent together as a family.

One of the highlights of our trip was a thrilling white water rafting adventure along the Verdon Gorge - an activity more dangerous to me than I realised at the time. The gushing waters and breathtaking cliffs that lined this spectacular river were a sight to behold. Adrenaline surged through our veins as the raft dipped, twisted, and turned, allowing us to embrace the exhilaration of this heart-pounding experience.

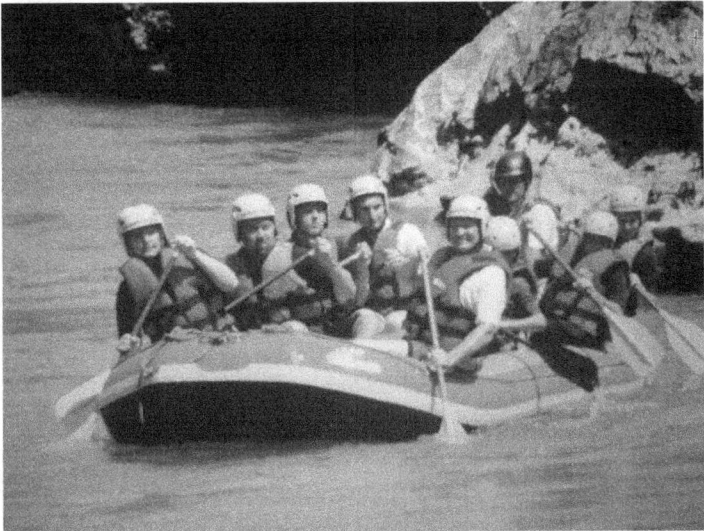

I'm on the far left and looking quite concerned

As the heat wave intensified, exertion in the scorching sun became increasingly taxing. What I initially perceived as the usual fatigue and discomfort accompanying extensive travel took an ominous turn. After the exertion of whitewater rafting and being dipped in the ice-cold river, the pain over my heart worsened, silently hinting at an impending health crisis.

With each passing day, the pain, to me at that time, was a signal, a warning 'gut feeling' that went unremarked amidst the excitement and adventure. Blinded by the allure of our surroundings and the immersive experiences, we carried on, oblivious to the ticking time bomb within my body.

Continuing our quest to explore the wonders of the French Riviera, we ventured to iconic destinations such as Monaco, St. Tropez, and Cannes. Monaco's opulence dazzled us as we marvelled at the grandeur of the Monte Carlo casino and the magnificent yachts docked in the harbour. St. Tropez captivated our senses with its vibrant atmosphere and dazzling beaches, offering a joyful escape from the daily grind. In Cannes, the town was abuzz with excitement, adorned with glamorous landmarks and the buzz of tourists relishing their retail therapy in luxurious boutiques.

It was a farewell to our French vacation. Still, the memories we had gathered during our time in France, despite the discomfort, would forever be cherished. The laughter, the breathtaking landscapes, the family bonding with Jason and Rachel. While our journey in France had both moments of pure joy and undesirable pain for my body, it ultimately served as a vivid reminder of the preciousness and fragility of life. Sometimes, amidst the most blissful experiences, hidden challenges await, silently reminding us to value our health and treasure every moment that we have.

Returning home, I continued consuming magnesium taurate supplements. It contributed to my overall well-being. The encounter with the French chemist, who generously shared his knowledge and expertise, underscored for me the importance of remaining open-minded and willing to embrace new ways of doing things in unfamiliar environments. The prescribed magnesium taurate supplements provided me with a lifeline.

Chapter 6

Relentless Struggle - Symptoms

As I reflect on the aftermath of the car crash, I can vividly recount the excruciating symptoms that plagued my every waking moment. My heart, once a steady beat that brought me life, had transformed into a relentless source of torment that defied explanation.

For three months after the crash, I could not lie down to sleep; whenever I went to lie down, the pain became so acute that I would immediately sit bolt upright again; sleep was achieved propped upright by pillows every night. Eventually, I became able to lie down again, but not on my back. I could sleep on my sides, but could no longer lie down comfortably on my back or my front.

Desperate for relief, I sought remedy with the expertise of numerous doctors. Every appointment afforded a glimmer of hope, as I believed they would finally unveil the root cause of my suffering. But time after time, my hopes were dashed as I found myself trapped in a disheartening cycle of misdiagnosis and dismissed symptoms.

One particular diagnosis stands out: fibromyalgia. After sending me for an MRI (Magnetic Resonance Imaging) scan and finding nothing in the result, my then GP attributed my agonising chest pain to this complex disorder and informed me that it was all in my head. As he started to write out his prescription, I declined it – I knew it wasn't what I had. It felt as though I was drowning in a sea of sadness and frustration, aching to be heard, understood, and ultimately healed. The doctors I had consulted had seemed unwilling to venture beyond superficial investigation.

Over time, I steadily delved deeper into the depths of my torment, desperate to unravel the puzzle that taunted me. Exhausted, I clung to the belief that there must be an underlying cause, a tangible explanation for the all-consuming anguish that had become my unwelcome companion. I refused to succumb to the notion that my suffering was merely a figment of my imagination.

The search for answers became my solitary mission. Medical records stacked up, each page fueling my disappointment as yet another door closed. But amidst the frustration and emotional turmoil, an ember of resolve burned within me. I knew I had to keep pushing and advocating for myself in a medical system that often dismissed the experiences of those who lived with unseen pain.

Days turned into months, months turned into years, and still, my heart continued to bear the weight of its invisible burden; but I was determined that a pivotal moment awaited me, a moment that would crystallise everything I thought I knew about my condition and present the opportunity for a breakthrough.

During this time, I discovered a strength I didn't know I possessed. It was a strength born out of a determination to overcome the greatest adversary I had ever faced – my own body. It was an emotional rollercoaster of not being listened to, the weight of constant disappointment, and the deepening sadness that accompanied my struggle.

In writing this little book, I wish to add my experience to the body of public knowledge, so that others who are still trying to solve their own puzzle may arrive sooner at a solution; to present possibilities for consideration, and to inspire the will to keep searching. With this stated objective, here are some of the symptoms that I experienced before being diagnosed, that hinted at the possibility of an aneurysm:

- The single biggest symptom was multiple episodes of deep vein thrombosis (DVT) in my left leg. A single DVT can be life-threatening. I have experienced deep vein thrombosis four times that I know of – mostly after undertaking a long-haul flight. Each time took from six months to two years to recover from and involved courses of the blood thinning drugs Warfarin and Heparin, with the associated prothrombin time tests to monitor my blood state. A DVT is extremely painful and long-lasting – it is more than enough motivation to wear compression stockings when travelling for long periods.

- Persistent and inexplicable chest pain, tightness, and discomfort.

- Shortness of breath and difficulty breathing, even during periods of rest.

- Intense and frequent headaches, often accompanied by dizziness or blurred vision.

- Strange bouts of fatigue, feeling excessively tired even with ample rest.

- Sudden and severe back pain, especially in my upper back.

- Waking up during the night with severe stabbing pains in my back in the region of my heart.

- Laryngitis - hoarseness and difficulty speaking clearly.

- Unusually rapid and irregular heartbeats (heart palpitations).

- Rapid blood pressure drops after a big meal.

- Sharp, shooting pain radiating down my arms and across my chest.

- Frequent bouts of dizziness and feeling faint, especially when standing up quickly.

- Persistent nausea and vomiting, without having eaten anything.

- Sudden changes in my eyesight, particularly double vision and loss of peripheral vision.

- Inexplicable numbness or weakness, particularly on one side of my body.

- Decreased coordination and difficulty with balance.

- Heightened sensitivity to light and sound causing sensory overload.

- Unusual mood swings, experiencing sudden bouts of anxiety.

- Difficulty concentrating and experiencing gaps in memory; manifest most often in forgetting words.

- Increased sensitivity to touch and temperature changes.

- Unexpected weight gain yet loss of appetite.

- Difficulty swallowing and a feeling of something stuck in my throat.

- Bending down and being unable to get back up due to extreme weakness or lightheadedness. I remember being in a newsagent one day and crouching down to see what was on the bottom shelf, only to find that I couldn't get back up again. I had to pull myself up on the magazine shelves to stand upright.

Please note that these signs can be indicative of various health conditions and should not be used for self-diagnosis. If you or someone you know is experiencing these symptoms, it is vital to seek medical attention immediately.

Even before my diagnosis, the persistent pain and discomfort had forced me to modify my habits. Things that I had taken for granted and had never thought twice about, became important or beyond my wherewithal. For example:

- Instead of jogging every morning, I switched to brisk walking to accommodate my physical limitations after the crash.

- I stopped waterskiing and swimming in deep waters and switched to shallow pools or supervised water exercises due to concerns about the impact on my health condition.

- As a safety precaution, I no longer used a hatchet to split logs for my fire. I started to buy them instead.

- I adapted my breathing techniques and started practising deep breathing exercises to manage anxiety and increase mindfulness – something I learned from competitive swimming when I was younger.

- To improve my well-being, I made changes to my diet based on food allergies or sensitivities, avoiding or limiting consumption of certain ingredients that used to trigger reactions.

- I became more mindful of portion control and adopted healthier eating habits, gradually reducing the intake of certain foods that had previously caused discomfort or negative reactions. I still put on a massive amount of weight in the 16 years since the crash though.

I had a noticeable difference in my blood pressure between my arms. This is known as inter-arm blood pressure asymmetry and can be an important diagnostic indicator.

When an aneurysm occurs on the aorta, it can affect the normal flow of blood through the arteries, creating imbalances in blood pressure. Checking the blood pressure in both arms is a straightforward and non-invasive way to detect this asymmetry.

To assess inter-arm blood pressure asymmetry, you can follow these steps:

1. Position yourself in a quiet and relaxed environment, sitting comfortably with both arms supported at heart level.

2. Use two blood pressure cuffs and place one on each arm according to the instructions provided with the blood pressure machines.

3. Inflate both cuffs simultaneously and then observe the readings when the pressure releases.

4. Compare the systolic (the top number) and diastolic (the bottom number) measurements between the arms to assess any significant difference.

Significant variations in blood pressure between the arms can serve as a potential red flag for an underlying issue, such as an aneurysm. It's important to note that inter-arm blood pressure asymmetry may also indicate other conditions like arterial disease or arterial blockage, so consulting a healthcare professional is crucial for proper diagnosis and further investigation.

Remember, this is just my experience of what I noticed in my body, and is not intended to replace professional medical advice. It's always best to consult with medical experts and research credible sources to ensure accuracy.

Chapter 7

Getting Diagnosed

It was in April 2016 when fate led me to the doors of the South West Acute Hospital in Enniskillen. My memory of the day I was diagnosed began with a stabbing pain in my back – I was spasming involuntarily with each shocking stab.

The day wore on, and the stabbing refused to relent. Helpless and scared, I found myself in the hospital A&E department, seeking respite from the persistent stabbing pain. With the evidence of my previous clots showing in my blood tests, the doctors decided to admit me for further examination as they thought I may have a pulmonary embolism (a blood clot in the lungs).

As I lay in the sterile hospital room, anxiously awaiting answers, my darling husband held my hand and never left my side. I have the most awesome husband and partner in life who truly believed my pain was where I said it was. The gravity of my situation began to sink in. The pain that had plagued me for years had led me to this moment, ensnaring me in its relentless grip. It was here, amid beeping machines and hushed conversations, that I sought both refuge and a solution.

Overwhelming desperation overtook me as I pleaded with the junior doctor standing before me, determined not to leave the hospital until the root cause of the stabbing pain was uncovered. No blood clot had been found and they wanted to send me home. The last place I ever wanted to be was a hospital, but I wanted even less to leave without getting to the root of it. Fortunately, my persistent plea caught the attention of a remarkable man, Professor Kelly, the Stroke Consultant.

With a flicker of curiosity in his eyes, Professor Kelly poked his head through the door, interrupting the conversation between the junior doctor and myself. Sensing the urgency and conviction in my voice, he inquired if the doctor had requested a CT (computed tomography) scan. Something deep inside me whispered that this was a turning point, a moment when the tides may finally shift in my favour. By this time, I had been admitted to the hospital and had already been in overnight. The CT scan was scheduled for that afternoon, renewing my hope for a definitive diagnosis.

The doctors ordered various additional tests, designed to unveil the darkest secrets hidden within my fragile frame. This was the pivotal moment that held the promise of answers; of a way forward where pain and uncertainty would no longer reign supreme.

My anticipation mounted as I was wheeled into the imaging room, engulfed by the sterile aroma that clung to the air. The mechanical whirring of the CT scanner became the soundtrack to my restless thoughts. With each passing moment, a tiny ember of hope flickered within me, for this machine held the power to reveal the underlying truth that had eluded me for so long.

Time wandered aimlessly as I anxiously awaited the results of the scan, the fear of the unknown casting shadows over my thoughts. Eventually, a pair of junior doctors returned to my room with the results of the CT scan. The scan results had been sent to the Cardiothoracic Department of the Royal Victoria Hospital in Belfast for analysis. No pulmonary embolism was found, but a 'dilation' of the ascending aorta had been observed. The junior doctors were unable to elaborate further on the significance of this. There was no mention of the word aneurysm.

That evening, Professor Kelly returned and we were able to ask about the significance of this discovery. Only then did the magnitude of the find become apparent. I learned then that this was what an aneurysm was. I had heard the word before but had never had reason to find out more about it. Shock, disbelief, and a newfound fear coursed through my veins as I absorbed this unexpected revelation. It was a bittersweet moment, for while the possibility of a clot had gone, it left in its wake the daunting reality of an aneurysm threatening to disrupt the rhythm of my very existence.

The hospital room, once merely a transient haven from my pain, now transformed into a battleground of emotions. Tears welled in my eyes as I gazed out of the window, my heart heavy with the weight of this newfound knowledge. In that profound moment, I whispered my gratitude to the doctors, the hospital, and the forces that led me here. It was in this unexpected turn of events that my journey truly began. With newfound determination pulsing through my veins, I steeled myself for the road ahead, resolute in my quest to reclaim my health.

Chapter 8

Finding a Surgeon

The South West Acute Hospital doesn't have a cardiothoracic department, so a solution would have to be found elsewhere. Ewan called our health insurance provider and started the process of making a claim. Having never had to use our health insurance before, this was new to us. It turned out that they had a dedicated cardiac team with a dedicated number for contacting them. Having collected all of the details of the diagnosis, they opened a new claim for us. They were then able to provide us with a list of consultants who perform surgery in this field, along with the contact details for each. It was then up to us to speak to them and identify a suitable candidate for the surgery.

As it turned out, it was my father who recommended to me the surgeon who ultimately performed my surgery. Quite where my Dad got the recommendation from, I'm not sure, but I did post-operatively discover that Mr Jones had been featured on a BBC TV series called 'Superdocs'. And a 'Super Doc', he most certainly is.

My husband contacted Mr Jones' secretary. She made an appointment for me to see Mr Jones, but advised that she needed a referral letter from my GP. The roadblock erected before me was a simple but frustrating condition — only those with a referral letter from a trusted doctor could secure a private consultation. My heart sank as the reality dawned upon me: we lived in the Isle of Man at that time and were only visiting Ireland to check on our property in Fermanagh when I was admitted to hospital. I had to return to the Isle of

Man, where a doctor, who had previously misdiagnosed me with Fibromyalgia, held the power to grant me the referral I so desperately needed.

Gathering my strength, I prepared for the emotionally draining task ahead. Boarding a plane, Ewan and I flew back to the Isle of Man, filled with trepidation and a flicker of hope that perhaps this time, my pleas would be heard. I was filled with anxiety as I sat in the waiting room, pondering my next steps. The same doctor who had repeatedly dismissed my concerns, telling me I read too many magazines, and attributed my agonising chest pain to the complexity of fibromyalgia, had shown little interest in unravelling the truth. His dismissive explanations left me feeling unheard and doubting my suffering.

With some nervousness, I described the symptoms and the diagnosis I received in the hospital in Enniskillen and made my request for a letter of referral. The conversation was strained and awkward. Self-doubt gnawed at my mind; was I asking too much? Would he belittle my concerns once again? Driven by my desperation, I navigated the minefield of the doctor's ego and carefully stated my case. In those tense moments, I silently begged for his understanding. After what felt like an eternity, he finally acquiesced, agreeing to write the coveted referral letter. Gratitude and relief washed over me, albeit tinged with a simmering mixture of frustration and disappointment. Why had I needed to fight so hard to be taken seriously? Ewan and I squeezed each other's hands with relief. As our meeting drew to a close, he asked me if I had any questions. I asked him what would happen if the aneurysm ruptured. He replied bluntly, "You'll die". He then recommended to us that we return to Ireland again as quickly as possible, as there was no facility on the Isle of Man to cope with my condition if I had an emergency.

Armed with a copy of the referral clutched gently in my hand, I retraced my steps, returning to Ireland with the letter Mr Jones' secretary needed for the consultation. Now resolve coursed through my veins; no longer would I allow doubt or dismissive attitudes to overshadow my quest for answers. Thank God for amazing men like my husband. You truly are a rock, Ewan. Little did I know that this would be just the beginning of a much more profound journey — a journey that would lead me closer to the truth about my health, and ultimately, to reaching the light at the end of a long, dark tunnel.

I first met Mr Jones on the 9th of May, 2016, three weeks after first being diagnosed with the aneurysm. In that time, I had undertaken a short round-trip to the Isle of Man and a longer round-trip to Germany; four flights in total. During our subsequent meeting, Mr Jones advised against air travel. He explained that the change in air pressure while flying increased the risk of clot formation. The flight Ewan and I had taken to Germany in particular had the potential to jeopardise my surgery due to the risk of developing a clot from the aneurysm.

This revelation occurred three months before my surgery. Suddenly, all of the DVTs after long-haul flights started to make sense. The car crash in 2000 had resulted in three broken ribs, one of which likely grazed the wall of my aorta, thereby causing a weakness. In the intervening years, this weakness would have steadily caused the aorta wall to bulge. I was at the root cause of the pain over my heart: an aneurysm on my ascending aorta.

It became a race against time. Mr Jones conducted blood tests to ensure that there were no additional risks or complications before my surgery. Connecting all of the dots to finally understand what had been going on with my body was a relief, but it was also suddenly much more frightening. The Time Bomb was ready to explode and I needed to keep relaxed, though the fear and upset of understanding it was making me the opposite. It was crucial to minimise any potential risks by staying in a relaxed state of mind.

Another CT Scan

The day after meeting Mr Jones, I attended the Kingsbridge Private Hospital in Belfast for another CT scan, this time tailored to Mr Jones' requirements.

The medical team guided me through the necessary preparations. A calm and reassuring nurse explained the process step by step, helping to ease my apprehension. After being fitted with a medical gown and an intra-venous line was set up, I was prepared to undergo sedation. When my turn for the scan came, I was wheeled into the CT room. The atmosphere was crisp and sterile, with various machines and medical equipment surrounding me. The radiology team attentively prepared for the procedure, ensuring that all necessary precautions and protocols were followed.

Despite the option to receive a sedative before the procedure, I declined, determined to face the scan with a clear mind. It transpired that this decision would later create a more impactful experience for me.

Lying on the CT table, the technicians meticulously positioned me in the proper alignment for optimal imaging. They explained that I would need to remain still during the procedure to achieve accurate results. The table glided into the machine, and a series of whirring sounds filled the room as the scan commenced. As the machine captured intricate images of my condition, a sudden blaring alarm filled the room. Panic ensued as an emergency team rushed in from all directions towards the machine I was in, quickly extracting me from its confines.

Confusion washed over me while I lay there, bewildered, surrounded by medical professionals. It was then that I discovered the cause of the alarm—my heart monitor had shifted on my finger. This accidental movement sent false alarms to the emergency team, triggering their immediate response. At that moment, the severity of my situation crystallised. The realisation hit me like a tidal wave - my aneurysm was not to be taken lightly. It was the first time the fragility of life became palpable, an ominous reminder that any moment could be my last.

Deeply shaken by this incident, I came face to face with my mortality, recognising the critical importance of my aneurysm's prompt repair. It was a sobering awakening, sparking a newfound awareness of the Time Bomb that lingered within, but also fueling my determination to confront my circumstances head-on.

The mishap with the sensor resulted in the scan having to be restarted. With my nerves shot, I had to be sedated. During the scan, I felt a profound sense of calm, even though unfamiliar sensations were occurring within my body. As I was told to breathe in and hold, a dye was injected into my bloodstream, which I could feel coursing throughout my body. It made me feel so warm and relaxed that I thought I had wet myself. The machine moved around me, capturing detailed images from various angles. The process was relatively quick, only lasting a few minutes, but it felt like a significant milestone in my journey. Afterwards, I apologised to the nurse, and said I thought I wet myself – to which she laughed and apologised for not warning me – it was normal to feel that, and she assured me that I hadn't.

Following the procedure, I was taken to a recovery area where I gradually regained full consciousness and alertness. The nurse closely monitored my vital signs to ensure I was recovering well from the sedation. Although I felt slightly groggy and disoriented, I was grateful for the reassurance and care provided by the nurse.

When the sedation wore off completely, I was provided with detailed instructions for aftercare and informed that the scan results would be forwarded directly to Mr Jones. Their analysis of the images would help determine the exact extent of the aneurysm and lay the foundation for the next steps in my treatment plan.

Leaving the CT room behind, I felt a mixture of relief and anticipation. Notwithstanding the abortive first attempt, the procedure had gone smoothly, and with those detailed images in hand, Mr Jones would soon be able to formulate a comprehensive and individualised approach to tackle the aneurysm.

Dr Donnelly, a Cardiologist at Kingsbridge Hospital, took time to discuss the CT scan and findings with my family and I. He began by explaining the complexities involved in treating this specific type of aneurysm. He explained that the ascending aortic aneurysm is located in a critical and delicate proximity to the heart, requiring careful consideration and expertise. Dr Donnelly elaborated, clarifying that this type of aneurysm necessitates a sternotomy as the method of access. This procedure involves dividing the sternum to access the thoracic (chest) cavity, providing the best access to repair the damaged section of the ascending aorta.

During his explanation, Dr Donnelly painted a comprehensive picture of the risks and benefits associated with open-heart surgery. He discussed the potential challenges, including the need for cardiopulmonary bypass, where a heart-lung machine temporarily takes over the functions of the heart and lungs during the operation. This process allows the surgical team to operate on a bloodless aorta, ensuring precise surgical manoeuvres while protecting the heart.

Additionally, Dr Donnelly explained how Mr Jones' surgical team would carefully repair the weakened aorta, utilising synthetic materials to reinforce and replace the damaged portion. He underscored the importance of performing such a procedure in a specialised and well-equipped cardiac centre like The Royal Victoria Hospital, where experienced surgeons like Mr Jones and dedicated support staff would be available for a successful outcome.

Throughout the discussion, Dr Donnelly demonstrated deep compassion and empathy, ensuring that my family and I felt supported and heard. He patiently addressed my concerns and answered questions, assuring me that this course of action was designed to minimise risks and increase the chances of a successful, long-term outcome.

By the end of the conversation, Ewan, Jason and I had a clear understanding of the necessity for a sternotomy to address the aneurysm. Dr Donnelly's detailed explanation instilled confidence, helping us to feel more prepared and involved in the decision-making process.

After we visited the clinic, we decided to treat ourselves to a well-deserved pizza at a nearby restaurant. It was a way to unwind and find some comfort amidst the overwhelming emotions that had been stirred up by the day's events. A nice Pizzeria with good food and wine was just what we needed.

As we sat down at a table, the aroma of freshly baked pizzas filled the air, instantly lifting our spirits. We found a moment of respite, engaging in light-hearted conversations and laughter that acted as a balm for our souls. The simple pleasure of biting into a slice of warm, cheesy pizza offered a brief reprieve from the weight of the day. We shared our thoughts and feelings about the medical procedure and the unexpected alarm that had disrupted the CT scan. We comforted one another, offering words of reassurance and support.

Chapter 9

What have Teeth got to do with it?

Early on in the process, Mr Jones imparted some crucial advice. He emphasised the importance of addressing any potential dental issues prior to surgery, including the removal of any problematic root canals or other dental concerns. This step was essential in minimising the risk of infections or complications that could potentially hinder the healing process.

Understanding the significance of this advice, I undertook to have my teeth thoroughly investigated. While my teeth may have appeared healthy by conventional standards, it was imperative to ensure that there were no underlying issues that could compromise my overall well-being during and after the surgery.

I want to take a moment to express my deepest gratitude to Dr Joe McEnhill of Belmore Dental Clinic in Enniskillen for the extraordinary effort he made to accommodate my urgent request before my surgery. His willingness to move mountains and make adjustments to his schedule to see me promptly was greatly appreciated. From the moment I reached out to Belmore Dental Clinic with my urgent need, Joe and his team sprang into action, ensuring that I received the dental care necessary before my surgery. This level of responsiveness and care surpassed my expectations, and for that, I am incredibly grateful. Not only did he provide me with exceptional dental care, but he also instilled confidence during what was a very stressful time. Getting the dental work completed was a pre-requisite for getting a date for surgery, so there was considerable pressure to complete it as quickly as possible.

Over multiple appointments, some stretching late into the evening, root canal treatments and other necessary restorations were undertaken, striving to eliminate any potential sources of infection that could have jeopardised the healing process post-surgery. Although minimally visible, the importance of this step could not be overstated.

Before meeting Mr Jones, I was unaware of just how significant teeth are as a pathway for infection into the body – in particular to the heart and brain. Achieving optimal oral health before my surgery highlighted for me the crucial role healthy teeth play in our overall well-being.

Ultimately, Mr Jones sought to maximise my chances of survival and ensure a successful outcome by removing the root canal dentistry and restoring affected areas prior to commencing surgery. The effort paid off, and my recovery was unmarred by complications or secondary infections.

It is always advisable to follow your surgeon's instructions and consult with them for further clarification or to address any additional concerns you may have. If you have a question, be sure to ask it.

Chapter 10

A Journey through The Royal Victoria Hospital

I entered The Royal Victoria Hospital on a bustling hot summer's day, with my husband Ewan and son Jason by my side. It was July 12th, 2016, which coincided with the band parades across all of Northern Ireland. It was the day before my scheduled surgery, allowing for important pre-operative procedures such as taking blood samples and general assessment of my health. Amidst the whirlwind of activities, I reconnected with, and was introduced to the remarkable individuals who would be pivotal in my journey - Mr Mark Jones, the Cardiothoracic Surgeon, Dr Suhaib Ahmed, the Assistant Surgeon and Dr Helen Gilliland, the Cardiac Anaesthetist. I offer my sincere apologies to the team members who introduced themselves to me, whose names I am unable to now recall. There was a lot to take in that day, and I was unable to take note of everybody's name. Their presence provided not only immense reassurance but also instilled confidence for a successful outcome.

I had researched all I could by searching online and reading many websites. I felt ready to go into theatre as I was aware of the journey I had to take. I had researched what a sternotomy involved, and understood in general terms how a heart-lung machine operated and its purpose. I had looked at the pictures, graphic as they are, and understood that the heart-lung machine would be used to temporarily take over the function of my heart and lungs, allowing the surgical team to safely repair the aneurysm.

I knew that Mr Jones would carefully cut out the damaged section of the aorta and replace it with a Dacron graft, inserted between the aortic arch and the aortic root; the graft serving as a permanent replacement to restore the normal function of my aorta.

Open-heart surgery with the aid of a heart-lung machine allows for a comprehensive repair of the aneurysm - so I learned through YouTube. It ensures the stability and durability of the graft, minimising the risk of rupture or further complications. While this approach typically requires a longer hospital stay and a longer recovery period, I felt I already knew I would have a speedy recovery as I was zoned into the whole procedure.

Had my aneurysm occurred on the descending aorta, there may have been the option of an endovascular repair, whereby a stent graft is inserted by making a small incision in an artery in the groin and feeding a small tube up the artery to the site of the aneurysm. The graft is then fed up the tube and installed inside the weakened area of the aorta. This procedure completely bypasses the need for the chest to be opened.

Overall, both endovascular repair and open-heart surgery are effective approaches to repair aortic aneurysms. The choice of procedure depends on factors such as the extent of the aneurysm and whether it is on the ascending or descending aorta, the condition and accessibility of the blood vessels, as well as the preference and expertise of the surgical team. In my case, Mr Jones said I had no option other than to have open-heart surgery.

Facing surgery with understanding, acceptance and inner peace.

As the morning sunlight trickled in through the window, my heart was heavy with a mix of emotions. Ewan and Jason reached out to me through FaceTime, their voices providing a semblance of comfort as they wished me well for the surgery ahead. Fighting back tears, I mustered all the strength I had, unsure of what lay beyond the operating theatre doors.

At precisely 8 am, a jolly porter named Billy arrived to take me to the theatre. Having already received a sedation pill from one of the nurses, I felt its calming effects beginning to soothe my unease. Trusting in the care and expertise within these walls, I surrendered myself to Billy's guidance as he carefully wheeled me down the hallway.

Throughout the journey, my thoughts drifted to the immense love and support I carried with me. Ewan, my doting husband, and Jason, my cherished son, had provided a comforting lifeline that connected us no matter the distance. Their tender words echoed in my mind, reminding me of the strength and resilience we shared as a family.

As we arrived at the doors of the operating theatre, I took a deep breath, allowing the light that surrounded me to uplift my spirits. With faith in the medical professionals, I gathered every ounce of courage and stepped into the realm of the unknown.

Within that theatre, a team of skilled individuals would work together with precision, expertise, and confidence born from experience. They would employ their years of study and training to bring me back to my loving family, who patiently awaited my safe return.

A wave of anxiety washed over me, engulfing my senses and leaving me feeling unsettled. Accompanying me was Dr Helen Gilliland, the Cardiac Anaesthetist who radiated compassion and competence. To alleviate my mounting nerves, she gestured towards the intricate array of machines and instruments that surrounded us, explaining their purpose and function. However, overwhelmed by the overpowering sights and sounds, all I could muster was a nervous plea: "Please, just take care of me, I would like to go to sleep now".

And so, enveloped in a blanket of trust, I surrendered myself to the capable hands of Dr Gilliland and her medical team. With their expertise and dedication, I knew I was in safe hands. It was time for me to let go, to embrace the peace that can only be found in the realm of unconsciousness.

Chapter 11

Recovery

The haze of anaesthesia slowly dissipated as I groggily regained consciousness. Perhaps unlike some people awakening from surgery, I had already subjected myself to countless gory and frightening YouTube videos, preparing myself for the various possibilities that awaited me. Yet amid all the fear and anxiety, one detail gave me a modicum of confidence: I was aware that I would wake up with a large tube in my mouth. As the fog lifted, my senses sharpened. The bleep, bleep, bleep of monitors and the faint whispers of medical staff punctuated the silence with rattling trolleys of different medical aids - blood pressure and body temperature machines with special little finger pieces - but through it all, I could sense that something obstructed my airway. Even before fully opening my eyes, I intuitively knew that the tube was responsible. Strange as it may seem, this foresight spared me from panic and allowed me to focus on what lay ahead.

Following the procedure, there were tubes and various wires connected to numerous machines and medications. Mechanical circulatory assistance during the surgery and post-operatively helped my heart provide the necessary cardiac output to sustain the pulmonary and systemic circulations. These were progressively removed as cardiac function improved. As I was able to breathe without assistance, ventilatory support was discontinued. Drainage tubes allowing blood and plasma to be collected from the chest cavity during healing were removed as the flow ceased.

The Cardiac Surgery Intensive Care Unit (CSICU) served as my sanctuary, where I received close monitoring from vigilant nurses. One nurse stood out with her vibrant purple hair. She was not only chatty and fun but also provided care on a one-to-one basis. Her expertise and attention to detail offered me a tremendous sense of security during those critical moments.

After spending two days in the CSICU, I was eventually transferred to the High Dependency Unit. Situated adjacent to the CSICU, this unit comprises eight beds and specifically caters to patients who no longer require assistance with their breathing through a ventilator but are not yet ready to return to the conventional ward setting. It provided me with the necessary transition period, ensuring sustained care and support as I moved towards recovery.

Recovering from surgery demanded both physical and emotional fortitude. The breathing apparatus became my constant companion as I fought to regain strength in my lungs. The process seemed never-ending, but I persevered, recognising that each breath marked a small victory in my battle for recovery. Gradually, I was encouraged to embark on short walks around the sterile, slightly overwhelming confines of the 5A ward. It was here that the importance of leg strength became evident. Every step I took, even with the assistance of monitors and hospital staff, felt like a monumental feat, but I knew that walking was crucial to rebuilding my physical endurance and reclaiming my independence. The post-surgery rehabilitation process demanded resilience, both physical and mental. It was an exhausting endeavour, encompassing a symphony of discomfort, pain, and frustration. But through it all, I clung to the belief that every hurdle crossed in this journey would inch me closer to reclaiming the life I once knew.

Perhaps the most crucial element in my recovery was the steadfast support of Ewan, Jason, Mum and Dad. From the moment I awoke in the hospital bed, Ewan and Jason's presence provided comfort and encouragement. Their kind words, gentle guidance, and reassurance served as constant reminders that I was not alone in this fight. My family became an anchor, tethering me to moments of strength and reminding me of the progress I had made. Their belief in my ability to overcome adversity infused me with further determination, strengthening my resolve to conquer each task at hand. Throughout the process, the challenges I faced felt immense. But as I reflect on those transformative days, I am reminded of the immense power and resilience hidden within each one of us. It is a strength that often lies dormant until summoned by adversity. And so, I continued to move forward, one step at a time. Drawn by the support of those who cared for me, I embraced the slow, steady progress, knowing that each breath, each step, held within it the promise of a brighter, stronger tomorrow.

I spent four more days in a private room in ward 5A under the care of the attentive hospital staff. This time allowed me to continue recuperating from the significant chest incision that had resulted from the surgery. Finally, with a deep sense of gratitude and relief, I was able to return home to fully recover and heal in the comfort of my own surroundings.

The Royal Victoria Hospital provided exceptional medical care, but it was the people within - the surgeon, the anaesthetist, the thoracic surgery team, and the diligent nurses - who truly made a difference in my journey. I am deeply grateful for their expertise, compassion, and commitment to my well-being.

My Dad's reassuring words offered comfort, easing the weight of uncertainty that had burdened me. As I embarked on my road to recovery, his calm and reassuring presence was a steady hand on my trembling shoulder, providing the confidence I desperately needed. Despite the countless times I sprayed him with my colloidal silver on the way home from the hospital, fervently trying to shield myself from infection, his understanding and patience never faltered. He traversed the roads of Northern Ireland, patiently driving me home, ensuring my safe return to the comfort of familiar surroundings, soaked to the skin with colloidal silver! (I make my own colloidal silver – it has anti-bacterial qualities, and I use it in a little spray bottle of water.)

As I gingerly stepped through the front door of our house after the journey from the Royal Victoria Hospital with my Dad, a mixed sense of relief and trepidation flooded over me. The hospital environment infused in every pore of my being was now an evanescent memory. Ewan travelled back from the Royal alone as I couldn't pull myself up into his 4x4 car. The corridors lined with bright white lights had been replaced by the comforting ambience of our own home. However, this familiarity came hand-in-hand with a newfound dependency on others. Simple tasks that once required minimal effort, such as lifting a kettle, suddenly transformed into eerie reminders of the weighty burden resting upon my healing body. "No heavy lifting," the wise words of Mr Jones echoed in my mind. Each movement became calculated, every gesture measured against the needs of a compromised body seeking recovery. The surgeons had wrapped wires around my sternum, holding my ribcage together as strength restored itself to weary bones. The knowledge that a wrong move could snap those delicate wires was an ever-present sentinel of caution, urging me to tread the waters of everyday life with the utmost care. The weight of caution hovered like a heavy fog in the air, contriving a meandering path that would lead me back to normality. Even mundane actions, like opening a drawer or pulling on a lightweight door handle, became moments of perplexity. Every pull felt like a delicate wrestling match within myself, as I weighed the consequences of exerting force against the precarious fragility of my mending chest. It was a frustrating and humbling realisation that recovery did not follow a linear trajectory; it danced on a precipice, asking for patience and dedication. The constant presence of Ewan amplified the poignant nature of my experiences. His supportive gestures, from acts of fetching cups of steaming tea to lending a sympathetic ear, reminded me of the resilience of the human spirit. It was through Ewan and Jason's collective love and steadfast companionship that I found comfort, and motivation in the journey toward complete restoration.

Each day unfolded with distinct challenges, but also opportunities for growth and surrender. The return from the hospital marked the beginning of a chapter dedicated to healing, strength, and resilience. It was a chapter filled with countless uncertainties, whispered hopes, and quiet victories. As I navigated the complexities of recovery, I clung to the support of my loved ones, gathering courage and determination to overcome every hurdle life placed before me. Ewan, thoughtful and caring, sought to assist in any way he could. Understanding the importance of maintaining a comfortable environment, he bought an air-purifying fan that tirelessly circulated fresh air. Its gentle breeze provided respite during a warm summer of resting in bed, cooling my weary body and soothing the discomfort caused by the healing process.

Six weeks passed since my surgery, and the time came for my check-up with Mr Jones. When we received the call from Mr Jones' secretary, a sense of nervous anticipation settled in the pit of my stomach. We entered his office and as we stepped into the room, the scent of antiseptic filled the air. The room seemed to be tinged with both uneasiness and a whisper of hope.

I anxiously awaited Mr Jones' arrival with Ewan by my side. The sound of approaching footsteps echoed down the hallway, followed by the characteristic creak of the door as it swung open. Mr Jones entered, his demeanour calm and composed, instilling a much-needed sense of confidence. Taking his time, he meticulously reviewed my medical file, studying every aspect of my case. Finally, after a careful and attentive examination, came the words that brought immense relief - "textbook success".

A rush of gratitude enveloped me as his words sank in. It felt like warm rays of sunlight breaking through a previously clouded sky. The weight of uncertainty began to lift off my shoulders, replaced by reassurance and a renewed sense of hope. At that moment, the significance of Mr Jones' expertise and the triumph of my recovery became undeniable.

As part of my recovery process, I was given a set of tools to aid in my healing. One of these was a lung exerciser puff, which I was instructed to use at home. The purpose of this device was to assist in expanding my lung capacity and promoting proper breathing techniques. As I held the puff in my hands and took the first inhalation, I could feel the controlled resistance building up within the device. Each exhale encouraged my lungs to strengthen and regain their full function. The regular use of the lung exerciser became an integral part of my daily routine, as I diligently followed the breathing exercises prescribed by my medical team.

In addition to the lung exerciser, another essential component of my recovery plan was a padded brace resembling a waistcoat. This brace served a crucial purpose - to keep my body straight and prevent any unnecessary movement of my bones, ensuring proper healing after the surgery. As I wore this brace day in and day out, I could feel its snug yet gentle support enveloping my torso. It served as a constant reminder of the delicate nature of my recovery process, and the importance of remaining cautious and committed to my healing journey.

If you have ever bought a car from a dealership, you may have been offered a special 'leaving the dealership for the first time' insurance policy, that covers you in the event you drive your new pride and joy straight into a fender bender. This is because those first few minutes of unfamiliarity with the vehicle and an over-abundance of caution with this pristine shiny new car make you more likely to have a prang. There should be a similar policy for patients recovering from major surgery.

Shortly after having my follow-up appointment with Mr Jones, I was having a small hay shed constructed. While outside speaking to the workman who was building it for me, I noticed a cable lying on the ground near where we were standing and thought that I had better move it before somebody tripped and injured themselves. As I lifted the cable, it dislodged a four-by-four post that was propped against a wall and sitting on top of the cable. The post fell in a scything arc and struck me right across the top of my forehead, opening up a long deep gash in my head. As blood poured from my head, I staggered to the house and called for Ewan. We pressed a towel to the gash to stem the flow of blood and then drove straight to A&E. I ended up with twelve stitches in my head, and a sobering realisation of how incredibly lucky I had been that it hadn't killed me. It was over-caution that got me hurt that day; tip-toeing around over-cautiously, instead of just being sensible and normal in my activities.

Despite almost cracking my head open, I made good progress with my recovery. As I followed the prescribed breathing exercises and wore the brace, I could feel a steady improvement in my lung strength and increasing stability in my body. Using the lung exerciser and the chest brace underscored the importance of actively participating in the recovery process, and reminded me that healing requires dedication, patience, and a willingness to embrace the necessary measures for a successful outcome.

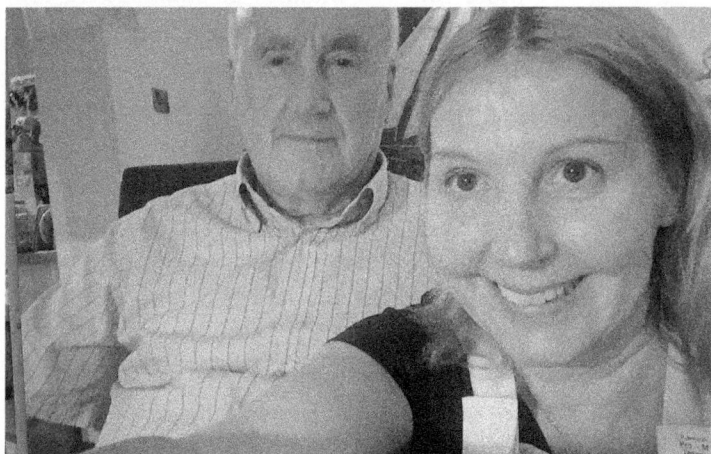

My Dad and I after he drove me home. Happily he had dried off from his soaking!

In every step of life's journey, there are guiding lights that illuminate our path, offering strength, support, and a love that knows no bounds. For me, a deep source of comfort lay in the enduring care and concern of my devoted parents. As I journeyed forward, the compassionate embrace offered by my parents held me tenderly, encouraging me to never lose sight of the love that had guided me so far.

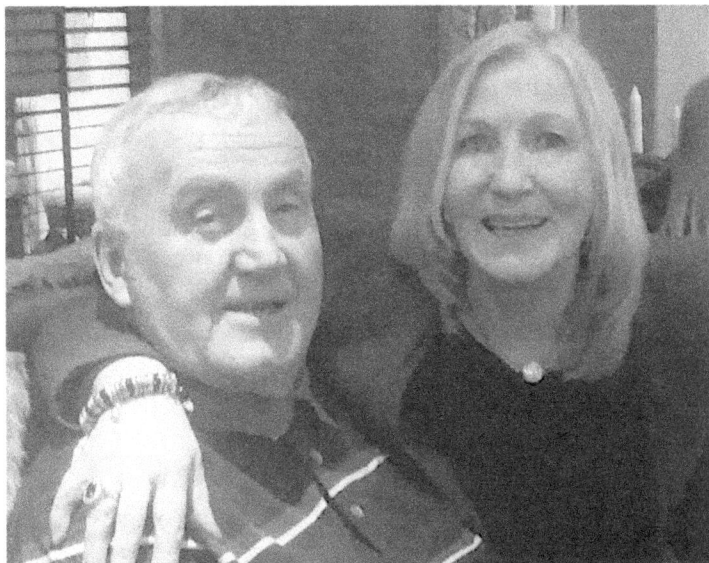

My dear Mum and Dad

Chapter 12

The Effects of Wire

Every step of the healing journey brought with it new challenges. While the surgery was a necessary step towards recovery, and I had read up on everything I could find to prepare myself for it, I didn't anticipate the pain and discomfort that would come from the wires that secured my sternum. As I learned, sometimes the road to healing can be fraught with unforeseen obstacles. In the months and years that followed my surgery, I found myself struggling with persistent discomfort.

All my life, I have reacted to jewellery made of nickel. Rings, earrings, bracelets – anything made of nickel would immediately cause my skin to develop a rash and then blister. It was only after the surgery that I learned that the 316L stainless steel typically used for the wires comprises about 10-13% nickel in its composition. Certainly, a much lower concentration than jewellery made of nickel would be, but had I researched this ahead of time, it is something that I would have discussed with Mr Jones. Just how much this may or may not have contributed to my discomfort is impossible to say, however, the rubbing that I experienced from the wires is not.

I discussed the matter of having the wires removed at my follow-up meeting with Mr Jones shortly after the surgery, but he told me that he would not consider removing them until at least three years after the operation. The wires that had been meticulously placed to support and stabilise my rib cage often brought me to the brink of despair. Their presence, intended to aid in my healing, became a source of excruciating pain. Once an ally in my recovery, the constant rubbing against my delicate bone had ignited a searing fire within, testing my emotional resilience as much as my physical strength. The pain, sharp and persistent, seemed to permeate every movement, turning even simple tasks into formidable challenges.

When the weather turned cold, the wire wrapped around my rib cage made me very aware of its presence. I could distinctly feel the freezing sensation penetrating inside my rib cage, akin to a frigid rod chilling me from within. This discomfort was undeniably intense, as the coldness seemed to seep deep into my bones, leaving me acutely affected by the icy touch within my body.

These wires are called sternal wires, they are commonly made of stainless steel and depending on the patient may range in number from 8 to 12 loops. The loops are closed and secured by twisting the tails together and laying the tail flat against the sternum. Depending on the surgeon, the wire tails may be laid pointing one way or another according to the 'Sternal Wire Code'. This code has been developed to provide a means of communicating to future medical investigators the nature of the work undertaken in the absence of medical notes. If employed, the code will signal its existence by pointing the top-most wire tail upward, to indicate the start of the code. Subsequent wire tails will be pointed downward to either the left or right of the patient's body. One loop for each graft present in the patient, pointing to the patient's left indicating a subclavian artery origin, or to the right for an aortic origin. The end of the code is signalled by another wire tail positioned upward. The wires and the code they spell out are clearly visible on x-rays, and so can be easily read non-invasively.

From what I can see in the x-ray of my own wires, this code was not employed by Mr Jones, so I have no notion that there was any discomfort arising from a signalling arrangement of the wire tails. Furthermore, since there was no message in the wires, there was nothing other than discomfort to lose in having them removed. I was determined that when the required three years had passed I would have them taken out.

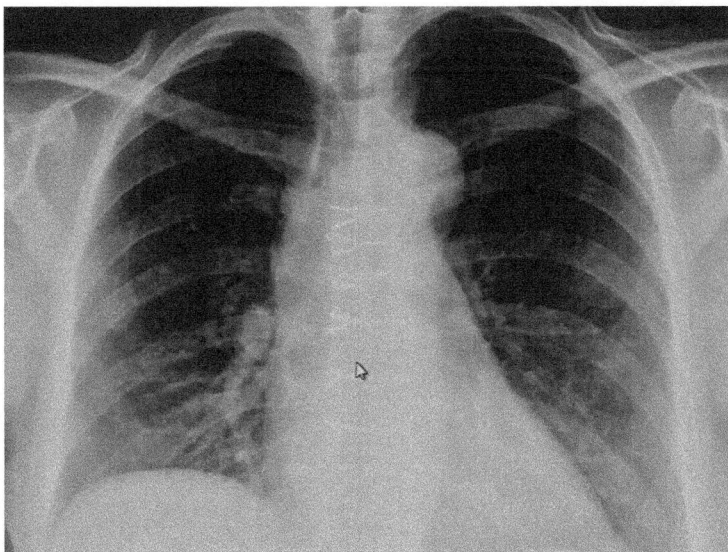

The sternal wires are clearly visible in this x-ray of my chest.

Chapter 13

Wires Removed

Booking an appointment with Mr Jones three years after my surgery, felt like a pivotal step towards reclaiming my health and obtaining relief from the ongoing pain caused by the wires. It was a moment tinged with both hope and anxiety, as I eagerly awaited the opportunity to gain clarity on my situation.

The anticipation weighed heavily on me as I sat in the waiting room, with my husband holding my hand. We were surrounded by people from all walks of life who, like me, sought answers and guidance from an expert in the field. The room buzzed with a mix of nervous whispers and gentle reassurances from loved ones who accompanied those seeking medical intervention.

Finally, my name was called by Mr Jones' secretary. I walked into the consultation room, my heart pounding in my chest, as I braced myself for the conversation that could potentially redefine my path to recovery. Mr Jones, with an air of calm confidence, greeted us warmly and invited us to take seats.

With genuine compassion, he listened intently as I recounted the excruciating journey of pain and inflammation brought on by the wires in my rib cage. He acknowledged how distressing it must have been and offered for me to be looked at by a nerve specialist. In response to my husband's question regarding the potential benefits of removing the wires, Mr Jones advised that it would not be beneficial. However, he provided reassurance that we would work together to explore alternative solutions to alleviate my suffering.

Examining the physical signs and carefully perusing my medical history, Mr Jones thoughtfully considered each detail. A glimmer of hope managed to break through the fog of despair that had consumed me for far too long.

Following a thorough examination, Mr Jones shared his theory that I may have developed an allergic reaction to the metal wires, a possibility that had not been considered before. His words carried a mix of validation and relief as if he had shed light on a mystery that had plagued me for three years after my surgery.

He explained the necessity of removing the wires to mitigate the detrimental impact they were having on my healing process. With surgical expertise and a compassionate tone, he assured me that this procedure was the best course of action to reclaim my health and restore equilibrium to my body.

We spoke at length about the potential risks and benefits of the surgery, ensuring that I understood each aspect of the procedure and its potential impact on my well-being. Through clear explanations and patient reassurances, Mr Jones alleviated any lingering concerns and instilled in me a newfound confidence.

As the consultation came to a close, Mr Jones informed me with a kindly smile that he would make arrangements for the wire removal surgery, and that his secretary would be in touch with the date. Three weeks later, I received confirmation that the surgery was booked for the 1st of October, 2019. Just before, as it turned out, the onset of the Covid-19 pandemic. It was as if fate had intervened, aligning the stars to favour my journey towards restored health.

Gratitude consumed me as I bid farewell to Mr Jones, his expertise and genuine care providing a ray of hope amidst the shadows of pain and hardship. With a renewed sense of purpose and a tingling anticipation in my heart, I embarked on the final leg of my long and arduous journey.

Chapter 14

A Memorable Surgical Journey

October 1st, 2019 Day of Wire removal.

After the consultation with Mr Jones, we returned home to the Isle of Man to wait and prepare for my important surgery. Five long weeks later, we flew back to Belfast, with excitement and a hint of nervousness, knowing that the wires that had been causing discomfort would finally be removed. Although short, it was a journey that would stick in our memories for years to come.

On the evening before my surgery, we met up with Jason to enjoy a casual yet meaningful evening out, sharing piping hot slices of pizza. As we sat around the table, I glanced at each beloved face present. Not only was my loyal husband sitting beside me, but my steadfast son, who was diligently studying at Queens University, had made it a point to stand by my side throughout this harrowing journey. Their reassuring presence infused the room with a palpable warmth, creating a sanctuary of comfort and courage amidst the sea of apprehension that had been swirling within me. In that precious moment, as the savoury aroma of cheese and tomato sauce wafted through the air, I felt wrapped in an embrace that words could never adequately describe. Ewan's strength, Jason's loyalty; their love, easing the burden of fear that had clung to my heart. Their steadfast commitment to uplifting my spirits and standing by me during this trying time embodied a level of devotion that transcended mere words. With each bite of pizza, laughter and conversation floating through the air, I couldn't help but be overwhelmed by a profound gratitude. Their presence and their fierce support not only bolstered my courage but infused me with a renewed sense of hope and resilience. What a fun way to enjoy the night before surgery. Thank you life.

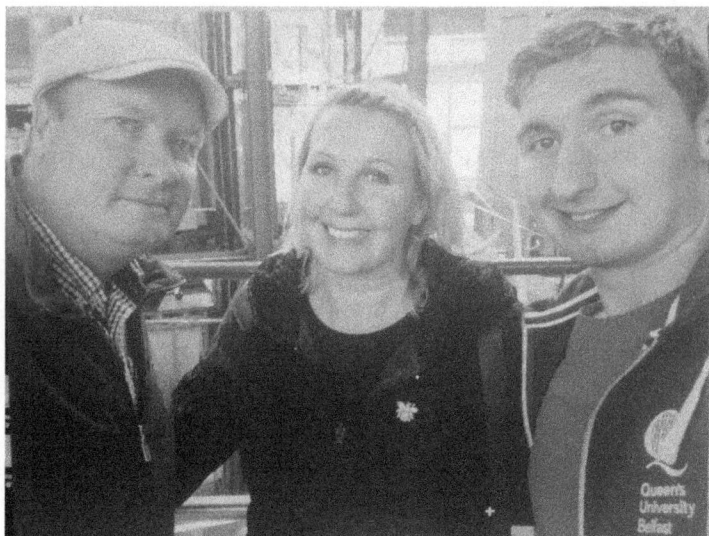

Ewan, Kim and Jason

The day of the surgery arrived, and I awaited my turn with a mix of anticipation and trepidation. It was in that lighthearted moment that I jokingly asked Mr Jones if he could perform a tummy tuck as well. He chuckled at the absurdity of the idea, knowing that it was merely a moment of levity in the face of a significant surgical procedure.

The procedure entailed removing wires from my sternum that caused me discomfort, which was substantially less invasive than my original aneurysm surgery. However, as I soon discovered, pain knows no logic or formula. Though the process was uncomfortable, I took comfort in knowing that I was under the care of a capable and attentive surgeon. The surgery left behind a scar of equal length to that of a major surgical procedure, surprising me with its fine and discreet appearance. More than just removing wires, this experience served as a reminder of the importance of having a supportive network in times of vulnerability. Ewan and Jason's presence at the dinner table the night before, and their support throughout the journey, were invaluable sources of strength and encouragement.

My journey to Belfast for wire removal carried with it unexpected moments of laughter, nervousness, and trust. It emphasised the importance of finding humour amidst pain and the profound impact of having loved ones by our side. This is a chapter of our lives that we will forever remember, and it serves as a testament to the power of resilience in the face of adversity.

The 1st of October, 2019, stands as a beacon of triumph and renewal, a date etched in my mind as the day I reclaimed my life from the clutches of pain. The surgery, expertly conducted by Mr Jones and his surgical team, removed the wires that had inflicted so much suffering, the metal that had once ignited inflammation now a distant memory.

Through their skilful hands and dedication to my well-being, I emerged from the operation with renewed vigour and a sense of lightness that I hadn't experienced in years. The wires, once agents of distress, had been vanquished, allowing my body the space and freedom to heal in its remarkable way.

As the world around me descended into chaos with the onset of a global pandemic, I found solace in my newfound state of health and an indomitable sense of gratitude. I realised that my journey, once shaped by pain and struggle, had been transformed into one of resilience, triumph, and a renewed zest for life.

Eight years after that initial significant surgery, I stand tall, once again a testament to the remarkable capacity of the human body to heal and rejuvenate. The wires, once a hindrance, can now only be seen through the lens of gratitude, for they pushed me towards a path of discovery and ultimately led me towards this moment of wholeness.

Since their removal, the previously described sensation of the cold rod inside my rib cage became even more pronounced in its absence, confirming that the wire was the exact cause of the chilling feeling. The newfound awareness of this connection highlighted the impact the wire had on my physical state, as the discomfort lingered for a while even after its removal, emphasizing the lasting impression left by their uncomfortable presence within my body

Amid uncertainty and struggle, the skill and compassion of Mr Jones guided me towards a brighter future, restoring my faith in the healing power of medicine and the dedication of healthcare professionals. With love and gratitude in my heart, I move forward with renewed strength, embracing a life brimming with health and possibility.

Chapter 15

A Wonderful Victory - Eight Years Later

As I sit here, reflecting on the incredible journey of the past eight years, it seems like yesterday that I faced a daunting diagnosis and a challenging path towards recovery. Today, I stand proud, not only as a survivor but as an advocate of aneurysm awareness. Every stage of my recovery brought me reminders of the fragility and preciousness of life. From the numerous doctor visits to the gruelling therapy sessions, each step was an exercise in being resilient and determined.

I also now have the benefit of hindsight. There are some things that I did right, some things that I could have done better, and some things that I did wrong. Let's start with what I got right.

Research. I did a lot of research before my surgery. This allowed me to prepare myself mentally for what I was going to undergo and to be prepared for my recovery. From the moment I regained consciousness, I was prepared for the tube that was inserted into my mouth. Had I not been aware of this ahead of time, the sensation of it could have caused me to panic and resulted in my remaining in Intensive Care for longer than I was. Your surgeon may advise you to avoid looking up the surgery on the internet, and if you are of a particularly squeamish disposition, this may be advice you want to follow. But for me, I benefited from having a clear understanding of what was going to happen, and what to expect. It afforded me the insight to have a meaningful conversation with my surgeon about how the surgery could be undertaken; how the incision could be effected to minimise scarring and so on. I did make some special requests, and he did oblige me with some of those requests, as far as surgical and professional protocol would permit.

Preparation for my return from hospital. I spent time before going into the hospital, preparing juices, soups and foods that could be frozen and available for me to use upon my return. I researched the fruits, vegetables and broths that promote healing, and I built up a stash of them ahead of time. Items that would be quick and easy to defrost and consume with a minimum of effort. This was time well spent and served me well as it turned out. I have included a list of the foods that I prepared in a later chapter of this book.

Returning from hospital. Ewan and I tend to occupy the extremes in whatever we do, and our cars at the time were no exception. I had a low-slung roadster sports car, and Ewan had a high off-road vehicle that required climbing up into. Neither of which was feasible for me to get in and out of immediately after my surgery. Recognising this weakness, my Dad drove me home in his normal height comfortable car. Such a simple thing, but had it not been recognised and anticipated, I would have been in a lot of pain, and risked movement in my sternum by trying to use one of our cars.

Silicone Skin. Silicone skin actively helps to reduce the redness of a scar by improving the skin's natural pigmentation process. The consistent use of silicone gel or sheets can lead to a noticeable fading of scarred skin, resulting in a more even and uniform complexion. The biggest relief I had from the silicone skin plaster was from the itchiness and discomfort: scars can become very itchy and uncomfortable during the healing process, and it's scratching them that can cause keloids to develop. Silicone skin acts as a protective barrier, shielding the scarred area from external irritants. It does not involve the application of chemicals or invasive procedures, making it suitable for individuals of all skin types and ages. It was a real lifesaver for my scar. The only downside to it is that it's quite expensive. I spun mine out by cutting the sheets into thin strips just wide enough to cover the scar area and no more. There's no point in covering skin that doesn't need it.

Mullein leaf tea. Mullein leaf is known for its anti-inflammatory properties, which can help reduce inflammation in the respiratory system. Inflamed airways can restrict airflow and lead to breathing difficulties. By reducing inflammation, mullein leaf can provide relief and support better lung function. It even tastes quite passable – it's very similar to green tea.

The value of thinking through the details of what you are about to undertake, and preparing accordingly cannot be overstated. If you think of the entire process as a job that has to be carefully prepared for and then flawlessly executed, you won't go too far wrong. As with most things in life, there is often only so much that you can realistically anticipate and prepare for, which is what brings me to the things that I could have done better.

Research. Yes, the same thing I mentioned above. I could have done more research and considered more fully the part of the process where they closed my sternum up, and the part of the process where I was recovering in hospital. This is where I took the most for granted and made assumptions. In particular, I wish that I had researched the methods used to reconnect the sternum and taken the opportunity to discuss this with Mr Jones. Wires are commonly used in effecting a closure, but they are not the only way. This is something that I would have benefited from exploring further ahead of time.

Clothing for recovery. One of the things that caught me out post-surgery, was the amount of swelling and inflammation that I would experience. This resulted in my pyjamas being too tight to be comfortable, and having to get Ewan and Jason to quickly go and buy some larger ones to give me relief. As any wife and mother will know, you don't send your husband and son to buy your PJs for you; what they will come back with is anybody's guess, and highly likely to be unwearable. I was lucky though – they brought back something serviceable, but I'll never wear those again!

Then there's the things I got wrong. It's one thing to take airline flights when you are unaware that you have an aneurysm, but it's another when you do. I could argue that I was ignorant of the risks associated with going up in a plane after I was diagnosed, which I was, but at the end of the day, I had sufficient information to have been able to make the connection with a bit of research. If reading this book is part of your research, then please make the connection now – don't fly until you get specific medical advice that relates to your particular condition.

Lifting. This is something that we all take for granted. Lift a full kettle, move a piece of furniture, pull a heavy door – all things that we all do without thinking about it. I got this wrong repeatedly when I left the hospital. Lifting any kind of weight exerts pressure on the body, both in terms of opposing the force of gravity and increasing the blood pressure demanded from the heart. Straining the body in this way after surgery is exactly the wrong thing to do. So lifting is out. Lift a half-filled kettle, not a full one, don't move the furniture, and get the door opened for you. If you are like me, and can't stand around idle while others work, this is going to take some getting used to.

I cannot stress enough the importance of listening to the survival signals from our 'gut feeling', or subconscious. Looking back on my life, I am inclined to believe that being in a state of peace has been instrumental in helping me navigate through the challenges of finding the source of the pain. After the car crash, I often said, 'I don't know why, but I can't do that' when confronted by activities that just didn't 'feel' right. I didn't know it then, but this instinct did protect me! That statement has now become 'I do know why, and I won't do that'. Aneurysms are no walk in the park.

Hindsight also now allows me to make the connection between the aneurysm and the multiple DVTs that I experienced. While deep vein thrombosis and aneurysm are distinct conditions, aneurysms can be the starting point for the development of blood clots that result in deep vein thrombosis. Consequently, I don't believe that it is a mere coincidence that all of the DVTs I experienced occurred after the car crash, or that they all occurred after taking long-haul flights. Looking at it now, I think it reasonable to conclude that the crash caused the aneurysm, and the aneurysm caused the clots. The long-haul flights simply acted as the environmental trigger that resulted in the clots being released from the aneurysm and travelling to my leg.

Eight years on from my initial diagnosis, I am 99% recovered from the aneurysm. The remaining 1% I have to attribute to the realities of having a graft. To this day, I am cautious about twisting my body too acutely – a simple action like turning to put on my seat belt in the car can kink the graft. The immediate result is a sudden surge of palpitations accompanied by a cramp-like sensation. This added layer of sensitivity makes me aware of the presence of the graft inside me and the care needed to avoid unsettling it. I learned that to unkink the graft and alleviate the palpitations and cramping, I have to shift and shuffle my body until the discomfort gradually subsides. This simple movement is a gentle and effective way to correct the kink in the graft and restore normal blood flow, ultimately relieving the palpitations and cramp-like feeling in my body.

The other consideration I have is lifting anything heavy. If I forget and I set about lifting something beyond my comfort zone, I end up with a pain in my chest and a raw feeling for the rest of the day. It's the kind of raw pain you get from a shoe that rubs a blister on your heel. The pain emanates from the area of the graft, so I can only conclude that it is not a good thing. So I avoid lifting anything heavy.

It has been a remarkable journey of transformation since the pivotal surgery back in 2016. The removal of the wire that had once caused me discomfort marked the beginning of a series of unexpected changes and incredible health benefits that have shaped the way I have experienced life in the years that followed.

One notable revelation post-wire removal surgery was the gradual but profound shift in my body's response to temperature sensations. The absence of the wire allowed me to feel the change as my real aorta membrane grew over the graft, creating a seamless integration that eliminated the contrasting feelings of hot and cold that once plagued me. For a long time, I could feel the 'gap' between the sections of the real aorta on either side of the graft as the blood passed through. As the years passed, this natural process of regeneration culminated in a state where I no longer perceive temperature changes with the same intensity. It is as if my body has reclaimed its equilibrium, and I find myself in a newfound state of harmony where the boundaries between external stimuli and my internal experience have blurred.

In the dawn of 2024, I stand here in awe of the immense changes that have unfolded within me. The graft that once stood as a foreign element has seamlessly merged with my own tissue, allowing me to embrace a sense of wholeness that transcends the physical realm. With the real aorta membrane as my ally, I am no longer just a sum of my parts, but a cohesive entity that pulsates with vitality and resilience. Moreover, the absence of sensation where the wire once resided is a poignant reminder of the body's remarkable capacity for healing and renewal. The gradual process through which my nervous system adapted and recalibrated itself speaks volumes about the innate wisdom that resides within us, guiding us towards a state of optimal functioning and well-being.

As I reflect upon this chapter of my life, I am filled with gratitude for the journey that has brought me to this moment. The challenges I faced along the way have become the stepping stones that propelled me towards a deeper understanding of myself and the resilience that resides within me. With each passing year, I find myself more attuned to the symphony of my body, harmonizing with its rhythms and rejoicing in the newfound sense of wholeness that now defines me. In my existence, the surgery of 2016 stands as a pivotal moment that not only healed my physical form but also ignited a profound transformation within me. As I look towards the horizon of endless possibilities, I embrace the future with a renewed sense of hope, knowing that the journey of healing and growth is a lifelong odyssey filled with infinite wonder and joy.

Chapter 16

A Gentle Voice in the Storm

It truly matters to have a strong team.

When the weight of fear pressed upon my weak frame, enveloping me in its embrace, he stepped forward. My dear husband, with his tender heart and caring soul, became my voice when I could no longer find my own. By my side, he wove a tapestry of courage and kindness, bringing narratives of wonder and adventure to life, lifting my mind far from the confines of uncertainty. In those moments of despair, when illness threatened to steal my joy, his soothing voice resonated through the room like a serenade of hope. With each turn of a page, he transported me to worlds where Swallows and Amazons roamed and swallows soared freely, allowing me to momentarily escape the confines of my physical pain.

As I lay there, bound by the limitations of my own body, his words became a beacon of light, guiding my thoughts towards horizons untrodden. His gentle cadence rippled through my weary mind, creating gentle pools of calm amid the turbulent sea of illness. Through the stories he read, he provided respite from the palpable fear and reminded me of the endless realm of possibility that lay beyond the confines of the hospital room. Imagination intertwined with gratitude, etching a vivid tapestry of appreciation for this kindhearted man who understood that storytelling had the power to heal, to mend emotional wounds, and to transform moments of despair into chapters of hope. His voice, like a comforting lullaby, harmonised with the rhythm of my breath, alleviating the sharp edges of pain and worry, casting them momentarily into insignificance. Each word he uttered was infused with the power to transcend the confines of my ailing body, nurturing the flickering flame of resilience within me. In those precious hours of shared tales, we navigated treacherous forests, danced with mythical creatures, and captured Captain Flint's ship. Each story unravelled a new layer of gratitude, affirming that my husband's presence was the greatest gift I could receive amidst the chaos of pain and suffering.

With my mind immersed in the stories and my eyes roaming the walls and ceiling, he transformed each corner into a realm of magic and enchantment. His reading became a lifeline, reminding me that even in the grip of illness and weakness, one's spirit can soar, finding comfort in the limitless realms of the imagination. Stories of innocence and simple adventure helped breathe life into my weary soul. With his soft voice and knowing smile, he shattered the confines of fear, creating an atmosphere of tranquillity within the sterile walls that surrounded us. As the sunlight danced gently upon our room, I thanked the universe for aligning our souls and intertwining our paths in such profound ways. He brought the gift of storytelling, artfully weaving words that nourished my spirit, fostering strength when my own was feeble.

Chapter 17
Animals Need Looking After

I am forever grateful for the love and support provided by my father-in-law and mother-in-law during my journey to recovery. They tended to my beloved horses, James and Monty, ensuring they were well looked after in my absence. While I fought my physical and emotional battles, they selflessly stepped in with no experience of handling horses, offering reassurance in the knowledge that my cherished companions were in their caring hands. Their dedication and genuine concern for my well-being was truly humbling.

To my father-in-law and mother-in-law: words can never convey the depth of my gratitude. Thank you for standing by me during this difficult time, shouldering the burden, and taking care of all the precious things that bring me joy. Your love and support are greatly appreciated.

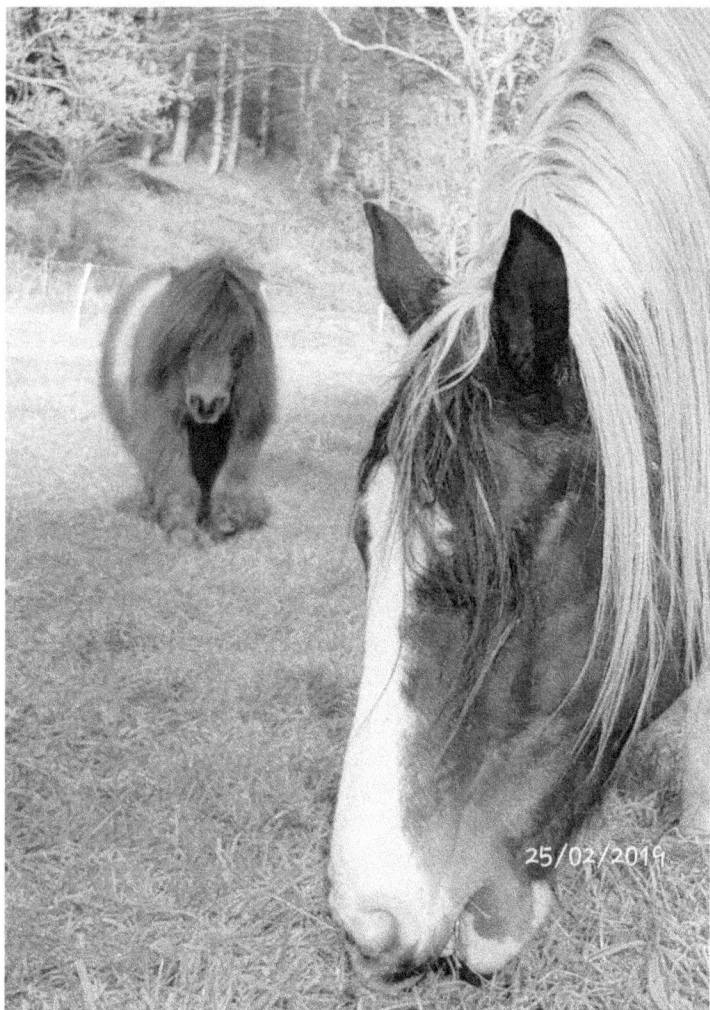

James with little Monty approaching

Chapter 18

Questions to Ask Your Surgeon

Here are 20 questions specifically for a replacement graft on the ascending aorta surgery:

1. What is the purpose of the replacement graft on the ascending aorta?

2. What are the potential risks and complications associated with this specific procedure?

3. Are there any alternative treatment options available for my condition?

4. How long will this surgery take, and what will be the estimated recovery time?

5. What is the step-by-step process of the replacement graft surgery on the aneurysm?

6. What are the expected outcomes or benefits of this surgery for my specific condition?

7. Are there any specific pre-operative preparations I need to make for this type of surgery?

8. Will I require anaesthesia, and if so, what type will be used for this specific procedure?

9. How many replacement graft surgeries on the ascending aorta have you performed in the past, and what is your success rate?

10. What is your plan for post-operative pain management?

11. Will I have any restrictions or limitations after the surgery, and if so, for how long?

12. What type of follow-up care or physical therapy is necessary for proper recovery after this surgery?

13. Are there any lifestyle changes I should consider post-operation to support the healing process of the ascending aorta graft?

14. Can this operation be performed with minimal scarring, or is there a possibility of having a discreet scar in this case?

15. Is there a potential need for a blood transfusion during the surgery, and can alternative methods be used to minimize transfusion requirements?

16. Are there any specific medications or supplements I should avoid before the operation related to an ascending aorta graft?

17. Will I need any medical devices or equipment after the surgery, such as a temporary pacemaker or support stockings?

18. Should I consider using silicone scar tape or any other scar management techniques to help optimize scar healing?

19. How long will I need to stay in the hospital after the ascending aorta graft surgery, and are there any additional costs associated with the hospital stay?

20. Is there a possibility of being allergic to the wire used during the surgery, and if so, can it be removed after the healing process?

Chapter 19
Recipes to Promote Healing

Here are some recipes for juicing or pulsing green vegetables and fruits, as well as a simple recipe for making bone broth on your return from the hospital.

You can freeze the prepared juices for convenience when you return home from the hospital. It's a good idea to pour the juice into airtight containers or zip bags, leaving some headspace for expansion during freezing. Label the containers or zip bags with the recipe name and date before placing them in the freezer.

When you're ready to consume the frozen juices, simply thaw them in the refrigerator overnight or place the container in a bowl of cold water to speed up the thawing process. Give the juice a gentle shake or stir before serving.

Juicing Recipes for Green Vegetables and Fruits:

1. Green Glow:
   - 1 green apple
   - 1 cucumber
   - 2 cups spinach
   - 1 lemon (peeled)
   - 1-inch piece of ginger

2. Cool Cucumber:
   - 1 cucumber
   - 2 celery stalks
   - 1 green apple
   - 1 cup kale
   - 1 lemon (peeled)

3. Popeye's Power:
   - 2 cups spinach
   - 1 green apple
   - 1 medium carrot
   - 1 small beet
   - 1-inch piece of ginger

4. Refreshing Green:
   - 1 pear
   - 1 cup kale
   - 1 cup pineapple chunks
   - 1-inch piece of ginger
   - Handful of mint leaves

5. Citrus Booster:
   - 2 oranges (peeled)
   - 1 grapefruit (peeled)
   - 1 cup spinach
   - 1 cucumber
   - 1-inch piece of ginger

6. Green Energy:
   - 2 green apples
   - 1 cup kale
   - 1 cup fresh parsley
   - 1 lemon (peeled)
   - 1 medium cucumber

7. Tangy Spinach Blast:
   - 2 cups spinach
   - 2 green apples
   - 1 lemon (peeled)
   - 1 medium cucumber
   - Handful of mint leaves

8. Pineapple Paradise:
   - 1 cup pineapple chunks
   - 1 green apple
   - 2 cups spinach
   - 1 medium cucumber
   - Handful of cilantro

9. Zesty Green Detox:
   - 1 green apple
   - 1 small beet
   - 2 cups kale
   - 2 celery stalks
   - 1 lemon (peeled)

10. Super Green Boost:
- 2 cups spinach
- 1 kiwi (peeled)
- 1 green apple
- 1 medium cucumber
- 1-inch piece of ginger

Simple Bone Broth Recipe:

Ingredients:
- 2-3 pounds of beef or chicken bones
- 1 onion, halved
- 2 carrots, chopped
- 2 celery stalks, chopped
- 4 cloves of garlic, crushed
- 2 tablespoons apple cider vinegar
- Salt and pepper to taste

Instructions:
1. Preheat your oven to 400°F (200°C). Place the bones on a baking sheet and roast for about 30 minutes until browned.

2. Transfer the roasted bones to a large stockpot and cover them with water. Add the onion, carrots, celery, garlic, and apple cider vinegar. Season with salt and pepper.

3. Bring the pot to a boil, then reduce the heat to low. Let the bone broth simmer for at least 6-8 hours, or even up to 24 hours for a richer flavour.

4. Skim off any foam or impurities that rise to the surface during cooking.

5. Once the bone broth has simmered for the desired time, remove the pot from heat and strain the broth through a fine sieve or cheesecloth to remove any remaining solids.

6. Bone broth can be easily frozen for future use. To freeze bone broth, allow it to cool completely in the refrigerator. Once cooled, transfer the broth into airtight containers or freezer bags, leaving some space for expansion during freezing. Label the containers with the date and contents.

If using freezer bags, it can be helpful to lay them flat in the freezer to save space and allow for quicker thawing later on. The broth can be kept in the freezer for several months.

When you're ready to use the frozen bone broth, thaw it in the refrigerator overnight or place the container/bag in a bowl of cold water to expedite the process. Once thawed, you can reheat the bone broth on the stovetop or microwave it before enjoying it. Remember to heat it thoroughly to ensure it reaches a safe serving temperature.

Remember to consult with your healthcare provider or a nutritionist to ensure these recipes align with your specific dietary needs.

Here's a grocery list for juicing recipes and a chicken bone broth recipe:

Juicing Recipes:

1. Fruits:
- Apples
- Oranges
- Lemons
- Berries (such as strawberries, blueberries, or raspberries)
- Pineapple
- Grapes

2. Vegetables:
- Leafy greens (such as kale, spinach, or Swiss chard)
- Celery
- Cucumbers
- Carrots
- Beets
- Ginger
- Parsley

3. Optional Additions:
- Chia seeds
- Flaxseed
- Turmeric

Chicken Bone Broth Recipe:

1. Chicken parts:
 - Chicken carcass or bones (preferably organic and pasture-raised)
 - Chicken feet or wings (optional, for added collagen)

2. Vegetables:
 - Onions
 - Carrots
 - Celery

3. Aromatics & Herbs:
 - Garlic cloves
 - Fresh thyme sprigs
 - Fresh rosemary sprigs
 - Bay leaves
 - Peppercorns

4. Optional Extras:
 - Apple cider vinegar (to help extract minerals from bones)
 - Sea salt or kosher salt (to taste)

Make sure to choose organic and fresh produce whenever possible. Adapt the quantities based on the number of servings you intend to make. Additionally, feel free to customize the ingredients and experiment with flavours based on your preferences.

Happy juicing and bone broth making!

Chapter 20

A Checklist for Your Hospital Bag

Here's a checklist for a hospital bag after major surgery; take into consideration potential swelling:

1. Comfortable Clothing:
- Loose-fitting button tops if scar is on chest
- Pyjamas
- Elastic-waist pants or shorts (to accommodate swelling)
- Non-slip socks or slippers
- Bra must be without underwiring – for comfort and healing

2. Toiletries:
- Toothbrush and toothpaste
- Face wash and moisturiser
- Body wash or soap
- Nail File
- Hairbrush or comb
- Shampoo and conditioner (if desired)
- Lip balm (I wouldn't be without it)

3. Personal Care Items:
- Glasses or contact lenses (if needed)
- Hearing aids (if applicable)
- Prescription medications
- Extra pillows for elevation and comfort

4. Entertainment:
- Books, magazines, or crossword puzzles
- Tablet or laptop
- Headphones

5. Electronics and Chargers:
- Smartphone
- Charger for phone, tablet, or laptop

6. Important Documents:
- Identification documents (ID, driver's license, passport)
- Health insurance card(s)
- List of allergies, medications, and any relevant medical information
(Have a family member take these things home when you are finished with them)

7. Comfort Items:
- Neck pillow
- Eye mask
- Earplugs (very important if you don't like noise)
- Stress relief items (stress ball, fidget spinner)

8. Extra Clothing:
- Underwear
- Extra pair of loose-fitting pants or shorts
- Extra comfortable tops or sleepwear

9. Personal Care Essentials:
- Menstruation products (if applicable)
- Hand sanitiser
- Facial tissues
- Wet wipes or baby wipes
- A facial mist toner to keep you cool and refreshed (Particularly in warm weather. I wouldn't be without it.)

10. Miscellaneous:
- Snacks that comply with any dietary restrictions
- Phone numbers of loved ones for easy communication
- Notebook and pen for jotting down any important notes or questions

It's important to note that each individual's needs may vary, so always consult with healthcare professionals or follow their specific recommendations.

Chapter 21

BallaBee

Once upon a time, in the enchanting countryside of Ireland, lived a woman named Kim. She possessed an artistic soul, brimming with dreams and emotions yearning to be immortalised on her canvas. On a serene evening, nestled within her snug room, aglow with the radiance of gentle candlelight, Kim excitedly suggested to her husband, "Let's paint by the flickering candlelight, and see what masterpieces we can create." Embracing the ambience, she found herself mesmerised by the vibrant colours of oil paints and a relaxing glass of red wine. Each stroke she delicately applied to the canvas reflected her deepest emotions, as she poured her heart into her artistry. Meanwhile, her husband skilfully painted a beautiful and colourful duck. As if guided by an unseen force, the colours took form, shaping themselves unexpectedly into a lively little bee, buzzing with vivacity and animation…...

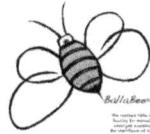

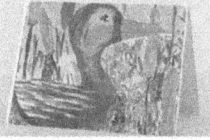

It wasn't until 2018, when we bought a property called Ballacuberagh, that I decided to name the bee "BallaBee." This name was inspired by the name of our new home, and the bee itself represents a delicate and beautiful soul navigating its way through life. Despite facing challenges, BallaBee serves as a reminder for me to maintain a positive outlook and to approach obstacles with a proactive spirit.

Through this symbolic creation, I found a way to playfully navigate life's journey and learn from each experience along the way. In creating BallaBee, I assumed the name as an alter ego for my creative output. The word 'Balla' is Manx Gaelic and means 'place of' or 'home of' and so BallaBee means 'home of bee'. Unlike wasps or other stinging insects, honey bees can only ever sting once. Being stressed to the point of stinging causes the honey bee to lose its life as the sting literally pulls its abdomen out. I recognise in the bee facets of my own nature - if ever threatened, I would instinctively react, even at the expense of my own well-being and life.

Despite facing challenges, I strive to maintain a positive outlook. Along my journey, I encountered some individuals who, though seemingly rude, served as valuable teachers, prompting me to respond not with anger but with a proactive spirit. It was from this blend of experiences that BallaBee came to life within me. Through this persona, I found a playful yet profound means to navigate life's paths with a proactive mindset and to glean lessons from each encounter.

I envisioned a powerful symbol of awareness for aneurysms. Through its adventures and interactions with others, BallaBee can serve as a reminder to prioritize health and well-being, encouraging proactive measures and screenings for aneurysms. As BallaBee encounters challenges and triumphs, it embodies resilience and determination, hopefully inspiring others to face obstacles with courage and positivity.

Chapter 22

Support

Ewan's observations

When Kim was diagnosed with an aneurysm, we were, as a couple, in uncharted territory. The learning curve was steep and immediate. The initial diagnosis was as a result of attending the accident and emergency department of the nearest hospital, but we had no idea who to go to to arrange the corrective surgery. Although we had health insurance in place, we had never had cause to use it before and were unsure of how it even worked. So I called them up and explained Kim's diagnosis to them. I was then put through to their dedicated cardiac team – a lovely group of ladies whom I would ultimately come to speak with many times. They opened a new claim for us and then explained which type of surgeon we would require for the surgery. I had never heard of a cardiothoracic surgeon before. I was provided with a short list of names and phone numbers for surgeons with the appropriate specialism, and it was up to us to make contact and arrange a consultation.

I set about calling the numbers that I had been given and was awaiting return calls when we got a suggestion from Kim's Dad. He gave us the number for Mr Jones at the Royal Victoria Hospital in Belfast. A call to Mr Jones' secretary got a swift response, and an offer of an appointment that same day. Unfortunately, it wasn't physically possible for us to get there in time, so we scheduled to meet him a few days later. The rapid response and the appointment at short notice were a huge relief. Getting to see an experienced and capable surgeon was our highest priority, and it couldn't happen fast enough.

In truth, nothing could happen fast enough for us. We soon found that scheduling appointments for scans, tests, evaluations and so on could easily stretch out months into the future if we let them. The time between being diagnosed and the surgery ultimately turned out to be three months, but it took a fair amount of persuasion and lobbying of the keepers of calendars and diaries to accelerate appointments and dates that would otherwise stretch off over the horizon. Exploring the opportunities for short-notice cancellations, and being flexible for appointments that were early or late in the day helped too. Getting a date for the surgery was like trying to nail a wave to the sand. It was third time lucky, as things turned out. We had two dates cancelled and surgery put back, as the hospital scheduling office juggled their varying demands. It seems that getting a theatre, and a surgical team to all line up at the same time is a more challenging matter than we had imagined it to be.

Managing medication was something that we had to get a grip on too. It is all too easy to forget when or even if a tablet has been taken, so we resorted to keeping a logbook together with the medication and scrupulously recorded what was taken and when. We also set alarms for certain times of the day, to ensure that the medication was taken at the correct intervals.

We went together to every appointment and stayed together as much as possible – with the obvious exceptions of scans and examinations – so that we had two sets of ears listening to everything that was being said. We prepared questions in advance of appointments and took them with us in a notebook so that we could write the answers next to them. It made things so much easier to recall afterwards when we were discussing the outcome of a consultation. Between us, we processed the information and thought of more questions to ask at the appointments, sparking off each other's avenues of investigation.

For all of our organisation and attempts at preparation, our focus was exclusively on Kim's requirements; it took Jason to think a bit wider and realise that there was no preparation made for our stay in Belfast while Kim was in hospital for surgery. For all that I had thought about it, he and I would have been sleeping in the car in the hospital car park! With no fuss or prompting, Jason organised hotel accommodation for us for the duration. Jason was a rock – we sat in the hospital canteen awaiting news of the outcome of the surgery, with the most dismal music playing in the background. It was Jason who comforted me as I cracked up with the overwhelming wait and the depressing music. Jason was a huge support to us throughout that entire period, and his calm zen-like disposition helped to keep us strong.

I read a good few books in those months. Many hours were spent in a dental waiting room while Kim had her teeth investigated and remediated before surgery. If you are going to spend your time reading while waiting, then be sure to read books that you won't mind being forever associated in your mind with a stressful period in your life. There are a couple that I wouldn't mind reading again – Erskine Childers' *The Riddle of the Sands* in particular - but I don't think I could read them without mentally placing myself back in that waiting room. Engaging novels that let your mind roam with the story being told are infinitely better in a waiting room than dry textbooks that struggle to hold your attention.

Reading to Kim proved to be quite therapeutic too. Jason and I took turns to read aloud while Kim recovered in the hospital. It took all of our minds off of where we were and why, and certainly helped the hours to speed by. We purposely read innocent adventures – Kim mentioned *Swallows and Amazons* as an example. Perfect escapism – nothing that reminds you of the realities you are dealing with at the time.

The hospital had fixed visiting hours, but because Kim was in a room of her own once she was out of intensive care, I found that I could stay with her around the clock. I wasn't hiding or staying in the room surreptitiously, I merely ensured that I got in nobody's way and gave no cause for the staff to ask me to leave. I can sleep anywhere, so an armchair in the corner was all I needed. Being there made the experience easier for both of us. We passed the time more easily together, and I was able to run errands for things if Kim had a need. It worked out well, and was quite unexpected that I would be able to do that.

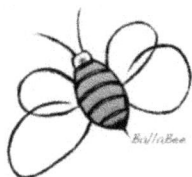

BallaBee Aneurysm Operation Preparation Notebook

This notebook, created in collaboration with Ballabee, is a companion for your journey after discovering you have an aneurysm. It includes helpful questions and memos to guide you through this challenging time. Let this notebook be your support system as you navigate the complexities of dealing with an aneurysm.

1. What type of aneurysm do you have?

2. Who are the key members of your healthcare team?

3. What are the treatment options available to you?

4. What are the potential risks and benefits of each treatment option?

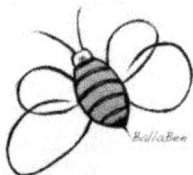

5. Are there any lifestyle changes you need to make to manage your aneurysm?

6. How often do you need to follow up with your healthcare provider?

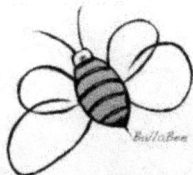

7. What warning signs should you watch out for that may indicate a complication?

8. Are there any restrictions on physical activity or other activities?

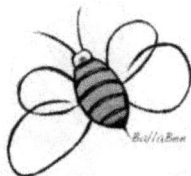

9. What resources are available to help you cope emotionally with your diagnosis?

10. Do you have a support network in place to help you through this journey?

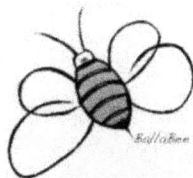

11. How can you communicate your wishes regarding treatment with your loved ones?

12. Have you discussed your wishes for end-of-life care with your healthcare provider?

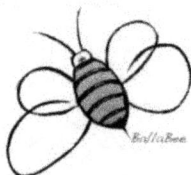

13. Are there any dietary changes you need to make to support your health?

14. How can you manage stress and anxiety related to your diagnosis?

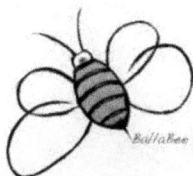

Bri/laBee

15. Have you explored any complementary therapies or alternative treatments?

16. What are the potential long-term effects of your aneurysm and its treatment?

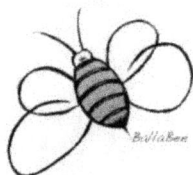

17. Are there any financial or insurance concerns you need to address?

18. Have you considered seeking a second opinion from another healthcare provider?

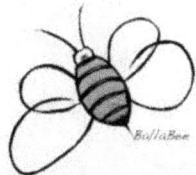

BullaBee

19. How can you stay informed and educated about your condition?

20. What are your goals and priorities for your health and well-being moving forward?

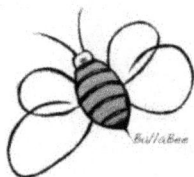

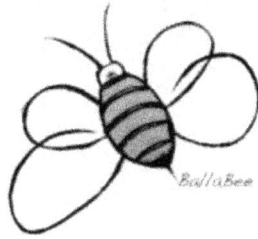
BallaBee

Just as being proactive instead of reactive can save lives in the context of human health, the same principle applies to bees. Ballabee, the proactive bee, understands that in its world, taking proactive measures is essential for survival. As bees are vital pollinators crucial for maintaining biodiversity and ecosystems, being proactive in seeking out nectar and pollen ensures their well-being and the health of their colonies. Reacting to changes, such as food scarcity or environmental threats, can have dire consequences for bees, making it clear that being proactive is key to their longevity and survival.

Notes

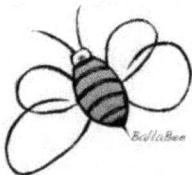

Notes

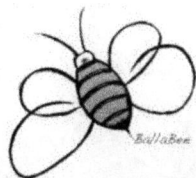

Notes

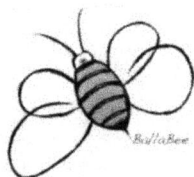

Notes

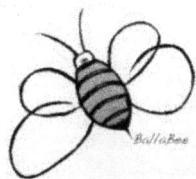

Notes

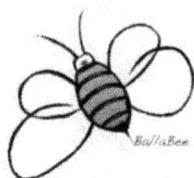

Notes

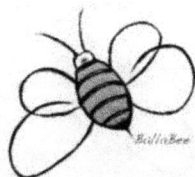

Notes

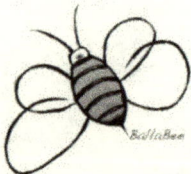

Notes

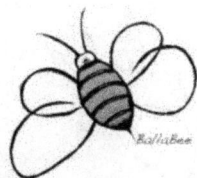

Notes

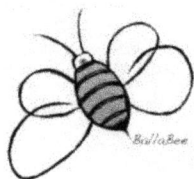

Notes

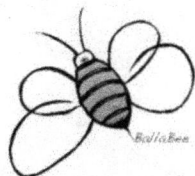

Notes

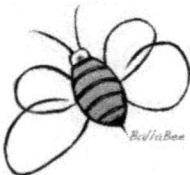

Time Bomb: A wake-up call for aneurysm awareness and mental health advocacy.

Notes

Ballabee's message: Act now, prevent the
sting of regret later.

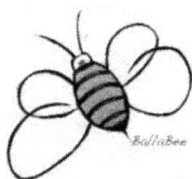

Notes

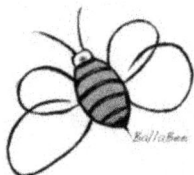

Ballabee Ltd: Planting the seeds of prevention, harvesting a healthier world.

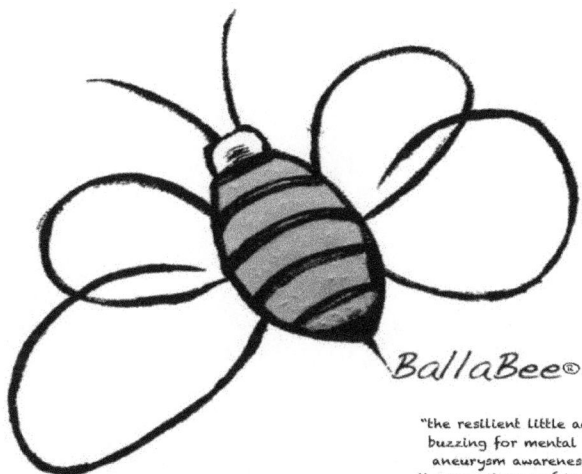

BallaBee®

"the resilient little advocate
buzzing for mental health,
aneurysm awareness, and
the importance of listening."

www.ingramcontent.com/pod-product-compliance
Lightning Source LLC
Chambersburg PA
CBHW031127020426
42333CB00012B/267